THE
KIDNEY DIET
COOKBOOK
FOR TWO

with **68** SIMPLE & DELICIOUS,
KIDNEY-FRIENDLY RECIPES
FOR TWO

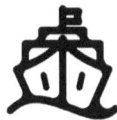

LASSELLE PRESS

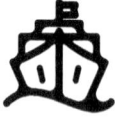

LASSELLE PRESS C<u>o</u>

ISBN-13: 978-1911364092
ISBN-10: 191136409X

CONTENTS

INTRODUCTION

Welcome!

Thank you for purchasing The Kidney Disease Cookbook For Two. If you are reading this then it is likely that either you or your loved one has been diagnosed with kidney disease at some stage. This can be a particularly daunting time for sufferers as well as their loved ones, but the good news is that, especially in the earlier stages of kidney disease, it is not too late to make simple changes to your diet and lifestyle in order to feel better and reduce the pressure on the kidneys.

This book aims to support you by outlining kidney disease and the different stages; providing guidance regarding nutrition for each stage of the disease; outlining hints and tips for cooking, stocking your kitchen and eating out; and lastly sharing over 68 perfectly portioned recipes for the two of you to continue cooking and enjoying together. Your diagnosis should not mean lonely dinners for one eating boring and bland foods: all of the recipes in this book are designed to be flavoursome, healthy and balanced meals that the two of you can continue to enjoy together. A complete nutritional breakdown of each meal is given, in order to allow you to calculate your daily intake and ensure you are sticking to the guidelines given to you by your doctor.

Finally, we wish you all the best along your journey with kidney disease and hope you find the information, guidance and recipes in this book helpful.

The Lasselle Press Team

I

KIDNEY DISEASE 101

If you have bought this book, either you or a loved one may be experiencing the symptoms caused by kidney disease. This chapter will outline the functions of the kidneys as well as some of the causes and symptoms of the disease. The good news is that if you are yet to suffer from the disease, or you're in the early stages, you can take steps to change your dietary and lifestyle habits in order to maintain healthy functioning of the kidneys for as long as possible. If you're at a later stage of kidney disease, you will have found that changing your dietary habits has become essential. This chapter aims to provide you with the information you will need to understand each stage of the disease.

YOUR KIDNEYS:

Despite their tiny size, the kidneys perform a number of functions which are vital for a body to function healthily. These include:

- Filtering excess fluids and waste from the blood,
- Creating the enzyme known as renin which regulates blood pressure,
- Ensuring bone marrow creates red blood cells,
- Controlling calcium and phosphorus levels through absorption and excretion

Unfortunately, when kidney disease reaches a chronic stage, these functions start to stop working. However, with the right treatment and lifestyle choices, it is possible to manage your lifestyle and continue living well, especially in the earlier stages of the disease.

CAUSES OF KIDNEY DISEASE

Unfortunately, 10% of all adults over the age of 20 will experience some form of kidney disease in their lifetime. There are a variety of different treatments for kidney disease, which depend on the cause of the disease. Possible causes are outlined below:

DIABETES: In the United States and other countries where the 'Standard American Diet' (discussed in chapter 2) runs rampant, the number one leading cause of kidney disease is high blood pressure and Type 2 diabetes. Both of these diseases are either completely preventable or at least treatable and once the root issue has been treated, kidney disease issues can also dissipate.

GLOMERULONEPHRITIS: Damage to the glomeruli (the filters in your kidneys), impairs the kidneys' ability to filter waste materials. This can be caused by damage to the immune system and if this is the case, can be treated with medication. It is either experienced for a short period of time (acute glomerulonephritis), or for a longer period of time (chronic). In chronic cases, further problems can arise such as high blood pressure, organ damage and later chronic kidney disease.

ACUTE RENAL FAILURE/ACUTE KIDNEY INJURY: Sudden damage or failure of the kidney can be caused by a rapid loss of blood to the kidneys, sepsis or even severe dehydration. Infection, poison and some medicines are also known to lead to acute kidney issues.

SUDDEN BLOCKAGE: Kidney stones, tumours, injuries and an enlarged prostate in men can stop urine from passing through the kidneys as it should. This can cause swelling in the lower extremities, a loss of appetite, vomiting or nausea, extreme tiredness, restlessness, feelings of confusion, or even an acute pain beneath the ribs (known as flank pain).

ECLAMPSIA: This can be experienced during pregnancy when the placenta doesn't function as it should do, creating high blood pressure and sometimes leading to kidney problems.

BREAKDOWN OF MUSCLE TISSUE: Under extreme pressure, for example when running a marathon or undergoing other feats of massive exertion, the body starts to break down muscle tissue after it has used all other available fuel. If this continues unchecked, too much of the protein known as myoglobin will ultimately end up in the bloodstream, putting undue strain on the kidneys and potentially leading to further implications.

IMMUNE SYSTEM: Common immune system diseases that can lead to kidney issues include lupus, hepatitis C, hepatitis B, HIV and aids. These can lead to what is known as chronic kidney disease (any form of kidney disease that lasts for three months or longer). Sometimes the sufferer of the immune disease will not experience the symptoms of the kidney disease until it reaches a chronic stage; this can be dangerous as it is a lot harder to manage once it has reached this level.

EXTREME URINARY TRACT INFECTIONS: Urinary tract infections that occur within the kidneys rather than the bladder are known as pyelonephritis and occur when a traditional urinary tract infection remains untreated long enough for it to spread into the upper urinary tract system. This can cause scarring in the kidneys which can lead to serious flaws in kidney functioning.

STREPTOCOCCAL INFECTIONS: Commonly known as a strep infection, this bacterium can infect the throat as well as various layers of the skin, the middle ear, the sinuses or even in a more severe case, a wide spread vicious rash known as scarlet fever. This bacterium is known to result in the glomeruli (individual filters in the kidneys) becoming infected.

POLYCYSTIC KIDNEY DISEASE: This kidney disease is typically passed down from parent to child and causes cysts filled with fluid to form on the kidneys themselves.

BIRTH DEFECTS: Depending on the severity of the defect, kidney disease could form simply because the kidneys do not function properly or because of an obstruction in the urinary tract before birth.

SYMPTOMS:

The symptoms of kidney disease vary widely and it is essential that you seek a professional diagnosis. Common symptoms below may be an indicator of the disease:

CHANGE IN URINATION PATTERNS: The most common indicator of chronic kidney disease; if you suddenly find yourself having to get up frequently at night to urinate or if the volume of urine passed significantly increases or turns pale, then you are advised to see a doctor. Likewise, if your urine becomes bubbly or foamy, contains blood, or significantly decreases in volume and turns very dark these ma also be signs that the kidneys are not working as they should.

SWELLING: Chronic kidney disease means that your kidneys can not filter waste materials or liquids properly and this can result in a marked swelling of the hands, face, feet, ankles or legs. This can be particularly uncomfortable for sufferers.

FATIGUE: Healthy functioning kidneys produce erythropoietin (the hormone that moderates the oxygen levels in the blood). The disease affects the kidneys' ability to produce this hormone, thus causing a lack of oxygen in the blood. With not enough oxygen reaching the brain or other muscles in the body, lethargy and fatigue is experienced. This is a form of anemia and can be extremely debilitating if not treated properly.

RASHES: A result of streptococcal infection as outlined in the causes section.

UREMIA: Bad breath which can smell of ammonia is sometimes experienced because of the waste materials not being filtered through the kidneys effectively. If suffering with uremia, people will often find that foods they are used to eating change in taste.

VOMITING OR NAUSEA: If left untreated, uremia can also lead to nausea and vomiting over a prolonged period of time . This type of vomiting is not usually treatable with common sickness medications.

BREATHING DIFFICULTIES: Excess fluid that cannot be filtered through the kidneys can travel to the lungs, making it difficult to breath. This can be especially problematic if experienced alongside uremia.

COLD SPELLS: Anemia can reduce blood flow to certain regions of the body and cause poor circulation. Circulation can become problematic as we age, gain weight or experience high blood pressure, however bad circulation is also a symptom of kidney disease and if you have experienced cold spells or flashes, this may be a sign of the disease.

DIZZY SPELLS: Prolonged anemia may also lead to frequent dizzy spells, making it difficult to concentrate on complicated tasks as well as impairing memory function.

LEG PAIN: Pain related to chronic kidney disease is actually felt in the kidneys themselves only a small percentage of the time. Leg pain is quite common as a result of swelling. Related issues such as bladder stones or infections as well as polycystic kidney disease are also known to cause pain in the sufferer.

5 STAGES OF KIDNEY DISEASE:

There are 5 stages of kidney disease which are measured by the glomerular filtration rate (GFR). This is calculated by a professional, according to the patient's serum creatine levels as well as their race, gender and age. The 5 stages and their characteristics are outlined below:

STAGE 1: People with stage 1 kidney disease will have some kidney damage though their GFR will remain in the normal range. During this stage doctors will work to determine the root of the problem so that it can best be addressed effectively. Those suffering from the disease are advised to keep their blood pressure lower than 130/80. Those who have diabetes are also encouraged to control their blood sugar levels. Regular checkups at the doctors are essential in monitoring the disease and its symptoms.

STAGE 2: By this stage the kidneys will have deteriorated further and the patient's GFR levels will be outside of the normal levels for those without kidney disease. At this stage doctors will determine how quickly the disease is progressing. Blood pressure and sugar intake guidance remains the same as at stage 1 and doctor visits should occur more frequently in order to keep a close eye on the symptoms experienced.

STAGE 3: GFR levels will have dropped significantly and at this stage doctors will start by checking for signs of additional complications including bone disease and anemia so that these can be treated accordingly. Monitoring check-ups will take place extremely frequently, if not daily.

STAGE 4: By this point, kidney function will have deteriorated further and GFR levels will have dropped dramatically. Doctors will very closely monitor the patient for potentially life threatening complications, and the available options (should the kidneys fail completely) are discussed and determined with the patient.

STAGE 5: Those with stage 5 kidney disease have an extremely low GFR level and will be experiencing kidney failure. Dialysis or a kidney transplant are the options for somebody with stage 5 kidney disease. At this point palliative care will likely be offered, depending on the pain, symptoms and side effects to the treatment given.

II
DIETARY CHOICES FOR A HEALTHIER LIFESTYLE

Your dietary and lifestyle choices can make a huge difference to your daily life, the symptoms you experience and in the early stages of kidney disease, the rate at which this develops. Changes can even prevent your kidneys from deteriorating, give you more energy, help you maintain a healthy weight, and prevent illnesses and infections.

Overall there are four main elements that you should be focusing on within your diet: phosphorous, potassium, sodium and protein intake should be limited and by making these changes in the early stages of the disease, you may even be able to prevent a far stricter diet in the later stages of the disease.

Unfortunately the diet many of us consume in the US and other western countries is not beneficial to our health. What nutritionists have termed the 'Standard American Diet' is unhealthy in many different respects: whilst including high levels of saturated fats, processed foods and animal fats, it is also light on complex carbohydrates, fiber, fruits and vegetables. All of this leads to a dramatically increased chance of stroke, heart disease, obesity, cancer and of course, kidney disease.

One of the main issues in this diet is the processed food, which is when chemicals have been added to food in order to preserve and make readily available to the consumer. In addition to these chemicals, processed foods include upwards of four times as much sugar as their natural counterparts. Excessive amounts of sugar increases the risk of type 2 diabetes, raises cholesterol levels, and creates a build-up of fat around the liver. As the liver works alongside the kidneys to remove toxins from the body, it is clear how these dietary choices can drastically increase the risk of kidney disease.

It is always best to consult your doctor and nutritionist to devise a meal plan specifically suited to your needs and the stage of the disease you are in. It is also important that you monitor and control your calorie intake as a loss of appetite is commonly experienced as a side effect of the disease and therefore weight loss needs to be carefully monitored.

HEALTHY DIETARY CHOICES

This section will cover the choices you can make to ensure a healthy diet and the best treatment for your kidneys. Advice and guidance will differ according to what stage of the disease you're in, however the principles remain similar throughout. Check with your doctor or nutritionist to ensure your diet plans are the best for you. Healthy food types and recommendations are provided as well as food types and groups to avoid or cut down.

CARBOHYDRATES AND FIBER: Although carbohydrates may be difficult to process when experiencing kidney disease at later stages, they do provide a vital source of energy that can combat the feelings of lethargy. As a low protein diet is recommended, carbohydrates can help to replace calories. Some carbohydrates are also fiber sources which in turn will benefit you in lowering cholesterol, losing fat and therefore reducing your risk of heart attacks. It is recommended that you eat at least 25 grams of fiber per day, even when suffering from stage 5 kidney disease and undergoing dialysis. You may become frustrated, trying to count your fiber levels as many high fibrous foods are also high in potassium, phosphorous and fluid (all things which are recommended to restrict on a diet for kidneys). Aim to eat foods that are high in fiber and try to limit foods high in potassium and phosphorus especially those that are not high in fiber.

FATS: Fats often get a bad name in society as we don't often distinguish between the healthy and unhealthy fats. Polyunsaturated and monounsaturated fats are extremely healthy when consumed in moderation.

If you are in need of extra calories because of a lack of appetite and weight loss experienced as a result of kidney disease, these types of fat are a good go-to as part of a balanced diet. Too much fat, particularly the bad trans-fats can lead to a rapid increase in cholesterol, increasing symptoms experienced as part of the disease and also increasing your risk of heart disease. This is in turn linked to diabetes and blood pressure, so it is always advised that you consume the healthy fats in moderation and steer clear of the unhealthy fats altogether if possible. Oily fishes like tuna, salmon and mackerel are excellent sources of these good fats. Choose oils for cooking and dressing such as coconut oil, canola oil and olive oil, rather than sesame or vegetable oils. Nuts and avocados can be consumed every now and then, but be aware of their levels of phosphorous and potassium.

PROTEIN: Although bodybuilders usually come to mind when we think of protein, it is actually an essential component of our diets and is vital for repairing tissues, keeping infections at bay and of course building muscle, even in the most exercise phobic of us! If you have chronic kidney disease in the first few stages, it is still okay to consume protein for up to 15% of your daily diet, with carbohydrates and fats making up the rest. This is the same amount recommeded for an average adult's daily intake. If your kidney disease has reached stage 4 then this reduces to 10%. During stage 5, and if you are on dialysis, the dialysis will filter out the waste toxins from your body as well as protein, therefore it is still crucial for you to include protein as part of your diet. Your dietician or doctor will advise on how much protein you should be consuming as at this stage it does have to be limited to approx. 1g protein per 1kg. body weight. Please always consult a professional for individual guidance.

PHOSPHORUS AND CALCIUM: Phosphates are salt compounds which include salt as well as other minerals; they work, as does calcium, to strengthen and keep our bones healthy. Extra phosphorous in the blood is usually removed by our kidneys, however kidney disease will prevent this process from functioning as it should. Unfortunately it's not as simple as just removing all phosphates from your diet as they are pretty much in most foods, but we can look out for those high in phosphorous. The food lists and guidance following, gives you a list of foods with low or medium levels of phosphorous as well as those to avoid with high levels of phosphorous. Typically stay away from processed foods as these often contain additives. Too much phosphorus can also lead to a calcium deficit which can lead to the extreme bouts of itchiness that many chronic kidney disease sufferers report. While annoying, the more serious issues if low calcium levels persist are pain, a general weakening of the bones, and even bone disease. A calcium supplement is recommended in order to counteract this if phosphorus levels remain too high. After this, medicines known as phosphorous binders may be required.

FLUIDS: As the kidneys start to decrease in functionality, the waste toxins and excess liquids are not removed from the body as they should be. This may lead to your doctor recommending that you limit the amount of liquids consumed, to take the load from the kidneys. Foods with high liquid contents also need to be considered as well as the drinks you consume, for instance fruits such as apples and pears, milks, soups, ice creams etc. This is more likely during the later stages of kidney disease and should be discussed with a professional.

POTASSIUM: A mineral that plays an essential role in keeping your heart healthy as well as regulating water levels in the body. Again, this is another mineral that is usually removed when in excess through the kidney filtration system. By now, you will get the pattern that too much of one particular mineral is problematic as the kidneys just cannot remove it in the way they can when completely healthy. That being said, extremely low levels of potassium are also harmful and kidney disease sufferers may experience either extreme. This is unique to you and your diagnosis, so will need to be monitored by a professional. Potassium is commonly found in many fruits and vegetables - stick with watermelon, tangerines, pineapple, berries, apples, cherries, pears, grapes and peaches.

IRON: Anyone whose chronic kidney disease has resulted in anemia will need extra iron in their diet. Options that are high in iron include iron-fortified cereals, kidney beans, lima beans, chicken, pork, beef and liver. It is important to discuss which iron-rich foods don't conflict with the other dietary guidelines with your medical professional or dietician.

STAGE SPECIFIC ADVICE

Your dietary needs and requirements will continue to change throughout the different stages of kidney disease and are subject to many different factors, therefore there is no blanket rule book for those suffering with kidney disease. The following guidance will give you a general idea of the key considerations and typical advice or recommendations given at the different stages. This should be used in conjunction with your healthcare professional and blood test results, in order to give you the best possible dietary guidance and treatment.

STAGE 1 AND STAGE 2: These stages are typically combined together because at this point the kidneys are still working at a similar level to healthy kidneys and symptoms may not be experienced yet. It is essential however at this stage to preserve as much of the kidneys' proper function as possible. This list below gives guidance on a variety of dietary choices that are usually recommended during these stages of the disease:

- Reduce dairy consumption in order to better control your protein intake.
- Increase your fiber intake by consuming more cereal, whole grains, vegetables and fruits.
- Eat more seafood and poultry than red meat.
- Baking, shallow frying in healthy oils, and steaming are better methods for cooking than deep frying.
- A maximum of 6oz. meat is recommended each day.
- Cut down or avoid processed foods completely.
- Keep alcohol consumption to a minimum i.e 1-2 glasses per week or none at all.
- Consume the recommended amount of calories for your height, gender and activity levels. Apps like myfitnesspal can help you calculate this.
- Use herbs and spices and balsamic vinegars to season your salads, vegetables and foods instead of salts and shop-bought salad dressings, which are usually high in preservatives and fats.
- Sodium: 1-3500mg. per day.
- Potassium: 2-5000mg. per day.
- Phosphorous - 1-1200mg. per day depending on weight.
- Protein - 0.8-1.2g per kilo of body weight.

STAGE 3: Primary goals in this stage include managing the levels of minerals and vitamins, hormones, fat cells, lipids and glucose. While some will need to focus on losing weight because of their fat cells, others may need to gain weight due to anemia or a loss of appetite. A dietician or doctor should determine the amount of calories you should be consuming each day.

- Limit or avoid trans and saturated fats. Replace with mono-unsaturated and poly-unsaturated fats.
- Fluid retention is not typically monitored during stage three, nevertheless, it is important to be aware of sudden swelling, weight gain, blood pressure spikes or urination issues as they can all indicate a decrease in the kidneys' ability to expel water.
- Vitamin D supplements may be recommended if you need to lower your phosphorous levels.
- Sodium: 1-3500mg. per day.
- Potassium: 2-4000mg. per day.
- Phosphorous - 1-1200mg. per day depending on weight.
- Protein - 0.6-0.8g per kilo of body weight.

STAGE 4: The quality of kidney functions will have been dramatically decreased at this point which is likely to lead to issues such as fluid retention, fatigue, trouble focusing, sleep difficulty, nerve issues, bad breath, abnormal tastes, loss of appetite, vomiting and nausea.

- Closely monitor and control potassium, phosphorous and sodium intake. The guidance will be specific to your needs and should come from a healthcare professional.
- Fluid retention varies from person to person during stage 4 depending on how well the kidneys are still working. Some type of fluid retention is almost always present, which is why it is important to monitor your fluid intake carefully.
- Sodium: 1-2500mg. per day.
- Potassium: 2-4000mg. per day.
- Phosphorous - 750-1000mg. per day depending on weight.
- Protein - 20-30g max per day.

STAGE 5: Many factors need to be taken into consideration at this stage when it comes to diet including response to dialysis, the likelihood of a transplant, your current nutritional concerns and your latest results from medical tests. Uremia during this stage makes it difficult for many people to eat regularly, which in turn brings on additional dietary concerns in terms of malnutrition.

- During stage 5 it is important to ensure that you are still consuming the recommended amount of vegetables, fruits and grains. Wholegrains and those high in potassium or sodium are to be avoided altogether.
- Cholesterol and saturated fats need to be cut out almost completely.
- Sodium intake will be extremely restricted at this point to help monitor fluid consumption.
- Calcium levels will be watched closely at this point as some people continue to need supplements while levels in others may return to normal (in which case calcium supplementation must be stopped).
- The amount of protein advised will likely be increased to counteract the effects of dialysis.
- Vitamin supplements for B,C,D and iron will all most likely be added to the diet to supplement the dialysis.
- Sodium: 1-2000mg. per day.
- Potassium: 2-2500mg. per day.
- Phosphorous - 7mg. per kilo of body weight.
- Protein -20-30g max per day.

III
EATING OUT AND SHOPPING GUIDE

It is a lot easier to stick to a healthy diet if you make the right choices on your grocery shops; keep the kitchen stocked with an array of healthy ingredients and you won't find yourself calling the takeaway or grabbing something on the go. That being said, eating out can be quite daunting. You don't want to miss out on spending time with your loved ones and doing the things you enjoy, but you worry about temptation or possibly causing a scene. This chapter will help you make the right decisions about what to keep in your kitchen as well as provide you with hints and tips on what to choose when you're out and about. Additionally, it is important to always read the labels and monitor the levels of potassium, sodium, phosphorous, protein and fats according to your needs.

KIDNEY SUPER FOODS

The following tables list a variety of food types and their dietary specifics. It is important to note that these are based on the given serving sizes and therefore, increasing the serving size will increase the levels of phosphorous, sodium etc. Stick to these serving sizes as one serving.

L= Low
(Potassium - Less than 150mg/serving, Phosphorous - Less than 150mg/serving, Protein - Less than 10g per serving, Sodium - less than 150mg per serving)

M = Medium
(Potassium - 151 -250mg/serving, Phosphorous - 151- 250mg/serving, Protein -10 - 20g per serving, Sodium - 150 - 250mg per serving)

H = High
(Potassium - More than 251mg/serving, Phosphorous - More than 251mg/serving, Protein -More than 20g per serving, Sodium - More than 251mg per serving)

Fruits 1/2 cup	Fiber	potassium	Phospho-rous	Protein	Sodium
Raspberries	H	L	L	L	L
blackberries	H	M	L	L	L
pears	H	M	L	L	L
apples cooked	H	L	L	L	L
apples raw	H	M	L	L	L
tangerine	H	M	L	L	L

Fruits 1/2 cup	Fiber	potassium	Phospho-rous	Protein	Sodium
strawberries	H	M	L	L	L
apricots	H	M = 1 apri-cot	L	L	L
blackberries	H	M	L	L	L
blueberries	H	L	L	L	L
lemons & limes		L	L	L	L
dried cranber-ries and cran-berry juice	H	L	L	L	L
grapes	H	L	L	L	L
raw fig	H	L	L	L	L
grapefruit	H	M	L	L	L
plums	H	L	L	L	L
pineapple	H	L	L	L	L
raspberries	H	L	L	L	L

Vegetables 1/2 cup	Fiber	Potassium	Phospho-rous	Protein	Sodium
peas	H	M	L	L	L
beans (green)	H	L	L	L	L
carrots	H	L	L	L	L
asparagus	H	M	L	L	L
cauliflower	H	L	L	L	L
cabbage (boiled)	H	L	L	L	L
broccoli	H	M	L	L	L
corn	H	M	L	L	L
eggplant	H	M	L	L	L
okra cooked	H	L	L	L	L
chickpeas	H	M	M	L	L
leek	H	M	L	L	L
cucumber	L	L	L	L	L
lettuce	L	L	M	L	L
onions raw	H	L	L	L	L
radishes	L	L	L	L	L
spinach	L	L	M	L	L
garlic	H	H	M	L	L
red bell peppers	H	L	L	L	L

Grains and other 1/2 cup	Fiber	Potassium	Phospho-rous	Protein	Sodium
flaxseed	H	L	H	M	L
barley	H	L	L	L	L
brown rice	H	L	M	L	L
cornflakes	H	L	L	L	L
corn grits	H	L	L	L	H
oatmeal	H	L	M	L	L
unsweetened cocoa 2 tbsp	L	L	L	L	L
wholewheat bread 2 slices	H	L	M	L	L
soy milk	L	M	L	L	L
pasta	H	L	L	L	L
tofu	H	M	L	M	L
1 rice cake	L	L	L	L	L
unsalted -almonds, cashews, hazelnuts, pine nuts, pistachios, walnuts, peanuts	H	H	H	H	L

Grains and other 1/2 cup	Fiber	Potassium	Phospho-rous	Protein	Sodium
lentils, white beans, soy-beans	H	H	M	M	L
wholegrain flour	H	L	L	H	L

Meat and fish 3 oz Dairy 1/2 cup	Fiber	Potassium	Phospho-rous	Protein	Sodium
feta cheese	L	L	L	M	H
brie cheese	L	L	L	H	H
duck	L	L	L	H	L
wholewheat bread 2 slices	H	L	M	L	L
chicken/turkey breast	L	L	M	H	L
beef - ground, sirloin, chuck	L	L	M	H	L
egg x 1	L	L	L	H	L

Meat and fish 3 oz Dairy 1/2 cup	Fiber	Potassium	Phospho-rous	Protein	Sodium
shrimp	L	L	L	H	H
cod/halibut/pollock/salmon	L	L	H	H	L
pork leg/chops	L	H	M	H	L
tuna, canned or yellowfin	L	L	H	H	M
greek/plain yogurt	L	L	M	H	L
milk skimmed	L	M	L	H	L
cottage cheese	L	L	M	H	H

THE SUPER FOODS SUMMED UP!

RED BELL PEPPERS: Red bell peppers are ideal for those suffering from chronic kidney disease as they are full of fiber, folic acid, vitamin B6, vitamin C and vitamin A while also being low in potassium. Another benefit for the kidneys is the high concentration of lycopene - an antioxidant that will increase kidney performance. Red bell peppers taste great in chicken or tuna salads or simply eaten with a low sodium dip. Roasted, they make a great addition to any salad or sandwich. They also add a mild kick to kebabs, egg dishes or as a part of a ground turkey or beef meal.

Red bell peppers contain approx. 10 mg of phosphorus, 88 mg of potassium and 1 mg of sodium per 1/2 cup serving.

CABBAGE: Cabbage contains high amounts of phytochemicals which break down toxins, improve cardiovascular health and fight cancer. What's more, cabbage is a great source of folic acid, B6, fiber, vitamin C and vitamin K while still being low in potassium. Cabbage is a great addition to fish tacos or coleslaw and can be microwaved, steamed or boiled depending.

Cabbage contains approx. 9 mg of phosphorus, 60 mg of potassium and 6 mg of sodium per 1/2 cup serving.

CAULIFLOWER: Cauliflower contains numerous compounds that help the liver remove toxins from the body. This will be a real benefit if the kidneys are struggling to do just that. It also contains lots of fiber, folate and vitamin C. Cauliflower is delicious with a simple dip, in salads, boiled or steamed. Cauliflower can be a great substitute for things like rice and potatoes and can be flavored uses herbs and spices and mustard.

Cauliflower contains approx. 20 mg of phosphorus, 88 mg of potassium and 9 mg of sodium per 1/2 cup serving.

GARLIC: Garlic is great to replace salt for flavoring and seasoning and it also naturally lowers cholesterol and mitigates inflation. Garlic has fewer anti-inflammatory and anti-clotting effects once it has been cooked so is best consumed raw for maximum results.

Garlic contains approx. 4 mg of phosphorus, 12 mg of potassium and 1 mg of sodium per clove.

ONION: Raw onions are low in potassium and high in chromium which is beneficial when it comes to helping the metabolism maintain its proper function. They can be consumed cooked or raw.

An onion contains approx. 3 mg of phosphorus, 116 mg of potassium and 3 mg of sodium per 1/2 cup serving.

APPLES: High in fiber and vitamin content which helps to mitigate inflammation. They are also known to reduce cancer risk, prevent heart disease, help with constipation and lower cholesterol. They are just as healthy cooked as they are raw and can also be consumed as a juice. Those who are monitoring their water intake should avoid apples because of their significant water content.

A medium sized apple contains approx. 10 mg of phosphorus, 158 mg of potassium and 0 mg of sodium.

CRANBERRIES: Cranberries are very acidic and help prevent harmful bacteria from forming in the bladder, which is great for avoiding infections in the urinary tract. They are also high in vitamins which can reduce the risk of heart disease or cancer. Cranberries are just as healthy when dried as they are when fresh and can be added to most salads or cereals for a delicious twist. Cranberry juice is also an option though those monitoring their liquid intake should consume in moderation.

Cranberries contain approx. 5 mg of phosphorus, 24 mg of potassium and 2 mg of sodium per 1/2 cup serving. Cranberry sauce contains 6 mg of phosphorus, 17 mg of potassium and 35 mg of sodium per 1/4 cup serving.

BLUEBERRIES: High in antioxidants, fiber and vitamin C, blueberries also help to mitigate inflammation. Their manganese content helps prevent bone related issues that may occur as a result of a calcium deficiency. Blueberries can be eaten raw, dried, baked, in a smoothie, or with cereal. Blueberries contain approx. 7 mg of phosphorus, 65 mg of potassium and 4 mg of sodium per 1/2 cup serving.

RASPBERRIES: Also high in antioxidants, these little super foods are known to help reduce cancer cells or tumor growth.

Raspberries contain approx. 7 mg of phosphorus, 93 mg of potassium and 0 mg of sodium per 1/2 cup serving.

STRAWBERRIES: High in fiber, manganese, vitamin C and other vitamins and minerals which are known to help prevent cancer, maintain heart health, and mitigate inflammation.

Strawberries contain approx. 13 mg of phosphorus, 120 mg of potassium and 1 mg of sodium per 1/2 cup serving.

CHERRIES: Eating cherries daily has been shown to measurably reduce the amount of inflammation that those experiencing chronic kidney disease experience. They are also high in antioxidants as well as phyto-chemicals which help reduce the risk of heart disease. Cherries are great on their own, in desserts and also as a sauce for either pork or lamb.

Cherries contain approx. 15 mg of phosphorus, 160 mg of potassium and 0 mg of sodium per 1/2 cup serving.

RED GRAPES: Red grapes get their color from the flavonoids they contain which help maintain heart health as well as reducing the risk of blood clots and improving oxidation and overall blood flow. They are also known to help reduce the risk of cancer and ease inflammation. Choose grapes the most vibrant in color. Frozen grapes taste delicious and are also thirst quenching, especially if you're having to control your water intake.

Red grapes contain approx. 4 mg of phosphorus, 88 mg of potassium and 1 mg of sodium in a half cup serving.

EGG WHITES: Egg whites are pure protein; they are also lower in phosphorus than egg yolks and they contain a wealth of vital amino acids. Egg whites can be eaten on their own, in salads, with tuna, or even in smoothies for those not on a liquid restricted diet.

An egg white contains approx. 10 mg of phosphorus, 108 mg of potassium and 110 mg of sodium and 7 grams of protein per 1/2 cup serving.

FISH: Besides being a great source of protein, fish is known to be an anti-inflammatory agent thanks to its omega-3 content. Those who have chronic kidney disease are encouraged to eat at least three servings of fish per week. Additional fats found in fish can help reduce the risk of heart disease as well as cancer. The healthiest fish in terms of omega-3 content are rainbow trout, herring, mackerel, tuna, albacore and salmon.

For example, 3 oz. of salmon contains 14 grams of protein, 274 mg of phosphorus, 368mg of potassium and 50 mg of sodium.

OLIVE OIL: Olive oil has been linked to a reduced risk of both heart disease and cancer. Extra virgin olive oil has higher levels of antioxidants than regular olive oil. It is a great choice for cooking, as a dip, marinade or dressing.

Olive oil contains approx. 0 mg of phosphorus, under 1 mg of potassium and under 1 mg of sodium in a single tablespoon

MUSHROOMS: Mushrooms contain more vitamin D than any other vegetable or fruit which helps improve kidney health. Mushrooms can be served in salads, soups, sides and as sauce for a variety of dishes.

An average medium white mushroom contains approx. 0 mg of phosphorus, 57 mg of potassium and 1 mg of sodium per 1/2 cup serving.

KALE: Loaded with flavonoids and carotenoids, both of which can reduce the risk of heart disease and cancer. Kale is also full of calcium, vitamin C, vitamin A and vitamin K. Kale is a great snack choice as it can be baked and consumed as a chip.

Kale contains approx. 0 mg of phosphorus, 0 mg of potassium and3 0 mg of sodium in a one cup serving.

SPINACH: The beta-carotene in spinach helps to keep your immune system as healthy as possible. It also contains folate, vitamin K, vitamin C and vitamin A. This is an ideal replacement for lettuce in most salads.

Spinach contains approx. 0 mg of phosphorus, 167 mg of potassium and 24 mg of sodium per 1 cup serving.

VITAMINS & SUPPLEMENTS: Vitamins and supplements that you would usually buy in shops should be avoided when on a renal diet as they may contain high levels that cannot be regulated by the kidneys anymore. Your healthcare professional may prescribe you a vitamin suitable for kidney disease patients, so please consult with them first.

FOODS TO BE AWARE OF

DAIRY: It is sometimes advised to limit your consumption of dairy whilst on a renal diet, this will help monitor your protein intake as well as control the amount of fat you eat. Try swapping full fat cheddars and parmesans for cottage cheese or brie.

CAFFEINE: Caffeine is a stimulant which makes it harder for the kidneys to filter. What's worse, consuming caffeine on an empty stomach has been linked to the formation of kidney stones and can also lead to an increase in calcium levels found in the urine. Try reducing the amount of caffeine you drink slowly; this will prevent withdrawal symptoms and ensure healthier functioning kidneys for longer. Green tea is great to swap for coffee and tea as its excellent qualities boost energy in the same way as caffeine does, making you feel great.

ARTIFICIAL SWEETENER: Avoid artificial sweeteners like saccharin and opt for stevia instead if you really need something to sweeten up your teas or meals.

SODA: Perhaps unsurprising as its main ingredients both make the list, soda is harmful to both your kidneys as well as your bones, in fact, drinking just 32 oz. of soda per day is known to measurably increase your risk of chronic kidney disease.

GMOs: Genetically modified organisms are likely to increase the number of free radicals present in foods; the chemicals and toxins in these foods cannot be filtered by the kidneys properly.

POTATOES: Sweet potatoes and white potatoes are high in potassium and therefore should be monitored if you're controlling potassium levels in your diet. That being said they can be leached by soaking in warm water or boiling twice to remove excess potassium and sweet potatoes in particular come with many other vitamins and minerals. Discuss with a professional for individual guidance.

TOMATOES: As above due to potassium levels. Canned tomatoes with no added salt or sugar can be consumed in moderation.

TIPS FOR EATING OUT:

Firstly, don't be embarrassed to make specific requests when eating out. Your health is more important than seeming to make a fuss and most of the time servers will be more than happy to meet your needs. If not, they're not worth your custom!

- Always ask for vegetables and side salads to be served plain and cooked dry without oils or butters.
- Avoid deep fried and breadcrumbed foods as these are often cooked in huge quantities of bad oils.
- When choosing steak, ask or opt for a smaller cut and have sides of vegetables, salads or suitable grains to fill you up.
- Seafood, chicken and turkey are better options but ensure they're baked, poached, steamed or boiled. If shallow fried, ask for them to cook this in olive oil.
- Try smaller or half portions if you're going to have a starter and a main.
- Ask for olive oils or vinegars on the side so you can control the amount you put on your food.
- Limit your alcohol intake and order a small glass. Ask waiters and waitresses not to top this up if you're somewhere fancy!
- Print the list of foods above or perhaps keep it electronically on your phone so you can easily check food types and opt for the best choice when dining out.
- If visiting friends and family members, share this list with them so they can make the best choices for everyone and not worry about whether they are doing the right thing.

IV
COOKING TIPS

So you've been diagnosed with chronic kidney disease and you know more about the symptoms, the different stages and the advised foods to try to eat more of and those you should consider monitoring or cutting out. This chapter will cover the best cooking methods when sticking to a healthy diet for your kidneys.

The guidance is much in line with other diets and healthy eating advice in general; cut out deep frying and instead try grilling, shallow-frying, steaming, roasting, poaching, broiling or baking. You can also try to limit sodium and potassium levels when cooking. Use healthy oils such as coconut or extra virgin olive oil as your main cooking oil and limit this if unnecessary i.e. for grilling, broiling or baking.

COMBATING SODIUM:

Salt is often over used to season our foods and act as preservatives in packaged foods. In fact, taste tests show that as little as one-eighth of a teaspoon is enough for most people to notice. Reduce the amount of salt you add to foods gradually and always check the labels of ingredients for their sodium levels.

If using canned vegetables, ensure the juice and broth has no added salt by checking the labels; fresh vegetables are always a better option. You can easily make broths and soups out of leftover vegetables or bones from chicken, turkey and even beef. See the recipe section for my favorite chicken stock recipe. Herbs and spices as well as balsamic or white vinegar can be used to replace salt when cooking or dressing foods. Sometimes, something sweet can be used for a surprising twist on your favorite meal, for example a squeeze of fresh lime or lemon juice. Likewise different cooking methods result in a variety of flavors from the same ingredients! Experiment with baking and roasting as well as grilling to liven up the same foods in the kitchen.

COMBATING POTASSIUM:

Boiling vegetables helps reduce potassium; if you've got extra time or you're really prepared, soaking them in warm water for a few hours helps this process. Cleaning and peeling potatoes and boiling twice is sufficient enough for stripping excess potassium out of the potatoes. When making stews and soups it is better to boil the vegetables first so as not to allow potassium to soak into the rest of the pot. If cooking with frozen or canned vegetables, they should be rinsed and soaked prior to use in order to reduce potassium levels. Low-sodium labelled products are not the ideal choice as these often contain other chemicals that are harmful to the body. Instead, use the methods described above to reduce potassium as much as possible and try using ingredients with a low potassium content where you can.

VI
GETTING STARTED

CONSIDER YOUR LIFESTYLE

Follows the tips below to make the transition to a healthy, kidney friendly diet as easy as possible.

- Eat a large breakfast, a medium sized lunch and a small dinner.
- Increase consumption of vegetables and fruits daily.
- Switch to olive oil based dressings.
- Try healthy snacks instead of quick and processed snacks e.g. roasted kale chips, plain yogurt, fruits and nuts in moderation.
- Eating smaller meals with a healthy snack in between will work for those needing to control calorie intake as well as those who have lost their appetite.
- Stay away from juices and sodas as they both contain high amounts of processed ingredients and sugar.
- Drink fresh water and green teas, but be aware of how much liquid you should be consuming each day.
- Don't eat after 8pm to allow your body and kidneys time to function before sleep.
- Find an activity or hobby to prevent boredom eating.
- Get into the habit of reading labels on foods and looking for sodium, potassium, phosphorous and calorie amounts.
- Eat a balanced diet to include protein, healthy fats and carbohydrates according to your diagnosis and personal needs. Apps like myfitnesspal help monitor the proportions of each of these through tracking what you eat daily.
- Stop smoking.
- Stay positive by asking friends and family members to try the healthy eating with you. That way you won't feel like you're losing out and you can still visit them without worrying about what you are going to eat.
- If you have a bad day, don't let it throw you off for good - we all have our bad days.
- Log your symptoms as well as what you eat in a journal every day or at least weekly if you can. This will help you keep track not only of how much and what types of foods you've eaten, but also of how they make you feel.
- Keep up with scheduled appointments and monitor your blood pressure to ensure it is not too high.
- If you're diabetic, ensure you monitor your condition and eat the right foods to prevent problems from escalating.
- Seek professional advice early as well as the support from loved ones. This can be an incredibly emotional time and you shouldn't have to experience it alone. Therapy might even be an option if you wish to talk about your feelings to a third party.

EXERCISE

The level of exercise you can safely perform while dealing with your chronic kidney disease will vary greatly depending on your current prognosis, the symptoms you are showing and your general level of physical fitness. Exercise is known to be especially helpful in the early stages of the disease and can help to fight off the initial feelings of fatigue that many people experience.

Exercise is useful for those who are looking to lose weight as a way to help mitigate numerous conditions that can lead to chronic kidney failure. Exercise can also strengthen the heart and is also known to help with anxiety as well as depression. For those who have to limit their fluid intake, strenuous exercise is not advised as you will become dehydrated and needing to consume higher quantities of water. In this case yoga and light walks are advised to keep fit and healthy whilst not exerting yourself too much. Speak with your healthcare professional for specific guidance.

Chronic kidney disease is a life-changing diagnosis, however there are ways of living with the disease and still maintaining a happy and healthy life. If you have been diagnosed in the early stages, further deterioration can be prevented and in all cases, living a healthy lifestyle and knowing about the right foods and drinks to eat will help you make the right choices in managing the disease and its symptoms. The recipes following are all created so that you can continue cooking and enjoying delicious recipes, whilst knowing that they are healthy and fresh options and are suitable for those suffering with the disease.

Use the recipes in conjunction with what has been recommended by your dietician or doctor acocrding to the stage of the diesease you are suffering. We wish you all the best with your cooking and the difference you make to your own life.

BREAKFAST

CREAMY CHIVE SCRAMBLE

SERVES 2 / PREP TIME: 3 MINUTES / COOK TIME: 15 MINUTES

A breakfast rich in iron and protein.

---

1 TSP EXTRA VIRGIN OLIVE OIL	2 TBSP ALMOND MILK
1/2 CUP RAW SPINACH	2 EGG WHITES
2 TBSP CHIVES, CHOPPED	2 SLICES MELBA TOAST
1 TSP NUTMEG, GRATED OR DRIED	

---

1. Mix egg whites, almond milk, nutmeg and chives in a bowl.
1. Heat a skillet on a medium heat and add oil.
2. Add the egg mixture to the skillet and stir for 5-6 minutes until eggs are cooked through and scrambled.
3. Now add the spinach and stir for 1-2 minutes or until spinach has wilted.
4. Plate up the melba toast and top with the scramble.

Per serving: Calories: 123; Fat: 8g; Carbohydrates: 7g; Phosphorus: 18mg; Potassium: 296mg; Sodium: 205mg; Protein: 6g

SPICY PEPPER & EGG TORTILLAS

SERVES 2 / PREP TIME: 5 MINUTES / COOK TIME: 15 MINUTES

A Mexican inspired breakfast for 2!

---

1 TBSP CANOLA OIL

2 CORN TORTILLAS

1/4 CUP RED ONION, DICED

1/4 CUP RED BELL PEPPERS, DICED

1/2 RED CHILI, DESEEDED AND FINELY CHOPPED

2 EGGS

1 LIME, FRESHLY SQUEEZED

1 TBSP CILANTRO, FINELY CHOPPED

---

1. Turn the broiler to a medium heat and place the tortillas underneath for 1-2 minutes on each side or until lightly toasted. Place to one side but keep broiler on.
2. Now heat the oil in a skillet on a medium heat and sauté the onion, chili and bell peppers for 5-6 minutes until soft.
3. Crack the eggs over the top of the onions and peppers and place skillet under the broiler for 5-6 minutes or until the eggs are cooked.
4. Serve half the eggs and vegetables on top of each tortilla and sprinkle with cilantro and lime juice to serve.

Per serving: Calories: 202; Fat: 13g; Carbohydrates: 19g; Phosphorus: 184g ; Potassium: 233mg; Sodium: 77mg; Protein: 9g

MEDITERRANEAN OMELETTE

SERVES 2 / PREP TIME: 5 MINUTES / COOK TIME: 15 MINUTES

A midweek or weekend breakfast treat.

---

1 TBSP EXTRA VIRGIN OLIVE OIL	1 TSP OREGANO
1/4 RED BELL PEPPER, DICED	PINCH OF BLACK PEPPER
1/3 CUP ZUCCHINI, DICED	4 LARGE EGG WHITES
1/4 RED ONION, DICED	

---

1. Heat olive oil in a skillet over a medium to high heat.
2. Saute the vegetables for 4-5 minutes.
3. Using a whisk, mix together the egg, egg whites, pepper and oregano together in a separate bowl.
4. Pour the eggs into the skillet over the vegetables and cook for 5-6 minutes until the edges begin to set.
5. Use a spatula to gently lift the edges of the omelette and turn over in the pan.
6. Fold the omellette in half and continue cooking for 3-4 minutes.
7. Remove omelette from the pan and cut in half to serve.

Per serving: Calories: 109; Fat: 7g; Carbohydrates: 3g; Phosphorus: 61; Potassium: 229mg; Sodium: 113mg; Protein: 7g

TASTY TOAST

SERVES 2 / PREP TIME: 5 MINUTES   COOK TIME: 10 MINUTES

The healthy version of this breakfast favorite.

---

2 EGGS

3/4 CUP UNSWEETENED ALMOND MILK

1 TBSP CANOLA OIL

2 SLICES WHITE BREAD, 3/4" THICK

---

1. Trim the crusts and slice the bread diagonally.
2. Lightly beat the eggs and add to the almond milk.
3. Pour oil into a skillet and heat over a medium heat.
4. Dip the bread into the egg mixture and add to the skillet for 3-4 minutes each side or until lightly brown.

Per serving: Calories: 109; Fat: 7g; Carbohydrates: 7g; Phosphorus: 83mg; Potassium: 97mg; Sodium: 120mg; Protein: 5g

OVEN BAKED PANCAKES & MIXED BERRIES

SERVES 2 / PREP TIME: 5 MINUTES / COOK TIME: 30 MINUTES

Mouthwatering morning pancakes!

---

2 TBSP COCONUT OIL

2 LARGE EGGS

1/2 CUP WHITE FLOUR

1/2 CUP RICE MILK (UNENRICHED)

PINCH OF SALT

1/2 CUP MIXED BLACKBERRIES, RASPBERRIES & BLUEBERRIES

---

1. Preheat the oven to 400°f/200°c/Gas Mark 6.
2. Add coconut oil to an oven proof skillet and place in oven until it has melted.
3. In a mixing bowl, whisk eggs until combined.
4. Add flour, berries, rice milk and salt and mix until smooth.
5. Remove skillet from the oven and immediately pour the batter into the hot skillet.
6. Place back in oven and bake for 25 to 30 minutes until pancake has risen slightly and is golden brown in color.
7. Plate and cut into 4 portions to serve.
8. Top with extra fresh berries to serve.

Per serving: Calories: 85; Fat: 5g; Carbohydrates: 8g; Phosphorus: 46mg; Potassium: 44mg; Sodium: 21mg; Protein: 2g

PEACH & BUCKWHEAT CEREAL

SERVES 2 / PREP TIME: 5 MINUTES / COOK TIME: 20 MINUTES

Nutritious and filling buckwheat porridge.

1/2 CUP PEACHES, SLICED

1/2 CUP BUCKWHEAT

1 TBSP HONEY

1 1/2 CUPS ALMOND MILK

2 CUPS WATER

---

1. Bring the water to a boil on the stove, add the buckwheat and place the lid on the pan.
2. Lower heat slightly and allow to simmer for 7-10 minutes, checking to ensure water does not dry out.
3. When most of the water is absorbed, remove from the heat and allow to sit for 5 minutes.
4. Drain any excess water from the pan and stir in the almond milk, heating through for a further 5 minutes.
5. Now add the peaches and honey.
6. Serve warm!

Per serving: Calories: 257; Fat: 5g; Carbohydrates: 48g; Phosphorus: 169mg; Potassium: 400mg; Sodium: 136mg; Protein: 7g

POULTRY

HOMEMADE HEALTHY CHICKEN STOCK

SERVING SIZE = 1 CUP / PREP TIME: 10 MINUTES / COOK TIME: 4 HOURS

This can be used in many of the recipes featured in this cookbook.

---

1 WHOLE ROASTING CHICKEN (AROUND 4-5LBS)	3 STALKS OF CELERY, SOAKED IN WARM WATER
3 CARROTS, SOAKED IN WARM WATER	1 TBSP EACH DRIED ROSEMARY, THYME, PEPPER, TURMERIC
2 MEDIUM ONIONS	1 TBSP WHITE WINE VINEGAR
4 GARLIC CLOVES, CRUSHED	11-12 CUPS WATER
2 BAY LEAVES	

---

1. Rinse off your chicken and place in a large saucepan or soup pan (remove giblets but don't waste them; add them in to your stock bowl!)
2. Chop your vegetables into large chunks (quarters at the smallest). Leave the skins on as they add to the taste and the nutrients - add to the pan.
3. Add the herbs, spices and pepper to the pan.
4. Fill your pan with water so that the chicken and vegetables are completely covered.
5. Turn stove on high and bring to boiling point before reducing the heat and allowing the stock to simmer for 3-4 hours.
6. Check at intervals and top up with water if the ingredients become uncovered.
7. Take off the heat and carefully remove the chicken, placing to one side.
8. You now need to strain the liquid from the stockpot into another bowl using a sieve to get rid of all the lumpy bits.
9. Leave the stock and chicken to cool.
10. Once cool, tear or cut the meat from the bones.
11. Once the stock has cooled to room temperature, add to a sealed container and keep in the fridge.
12. Save the chicken for a delicious salad or to add back into the stock to make a chunky chicken soup.
13. The stock can be kept for 3 days in the fridge/3 months in freezer in an airtight Tupperware box or Kilner jar - just skim off the fat when ready to use.

Per serving: Calories: 40; Fat: 2; Carbohydrates: 3; Phosphorus: 80; Potassium: 170; Sodium: 72; Protein: 5

STUFFED BELL PEPPERS

SERVES 2 / PREP TIME: 5 MINUTES / COOK TIME: 40 MINUTES

Turkey and couscous filled peppers.

---

2 LARGE GREEN BELL PEPPERS, CUT IN HALF

5 OZ LEAN GROUND TURKEY

1 CUP COOKED COUSCOUS

1 TBSP CAYENNE PEPPER

1 TBSP PARSLEY

1 TSP BLACK PEPPER

1/2 RED ONION, FINELY DICED

1 CLOVE GARLIC, MINCED

1 LIME

---

1. Preheat the oven to 350°f/170°c/Gas Mark 4.
2. Remove seeds from the middle of the bell peppers and layer onto a baking tray.
3. Combine the turkey mince with the onion, garlic, herbs and spices and stuff the peppers with the mixture.
4. Add to the oven for 30-40 minutes or until turkey is cooked through.
5. Serve with a side of couscous and a squeeze of fresh lime.

Per serving: Calories: 277; Fat: 4g; Carbohydrates: 28g; Phosphorus: 225mg; Potassium: 300mg; Sodium: 60mg; Protein: 24g

HOMEMADE JERK CHICKEN

SERVES 2 / PREP TIME: 5 MINUTES / COOK TIME: 40 MINUTES

Enjoy the taste of the Caribbean.

2X 3OZ SKINLESS CHICKEN BREASTS	1 TSP THYME
1 TSP OLIVE OIL	1 TSP CINAMMON
1 TSP NUTMEG	1 TBSP ALLSPICE
1 TSP CURRY POWDER	1/2 LIME
1/2 GARLIC CLOVE, MINCED	1/2 CUP WILD RICE
1 TSP GINGER, MINCED	1/4 CUP FRESH GREEN PEAS
1 TSP CAYENNE PEPPER	

---

1. Preheat the oven to 350°f/170°c/Gas Mark 4.
2. Prepare marinade by mixing olive oil and all of the spices.
3. Pour the marinade over the chicken in a baking dish and place in oven for 35-40 minutes. (You could leave this in the refridgerator over night for more flavor!)
4. Meanwhile prepare your rice by bringing a pan of water to the boil, add rice and cover and simmer for 20 minutes. Add the peas to the pan in the last 5 minutes of cooking time.
5. Drain and cover the rice and return to the stove for 5 minutes.
6. When chicken is cooked through, serve on a bed of rice and peas and squeeze fresh lime juice over the top.
7. Enjoy.

Per serving: Calories: 293; Fat: 10; Carbohydrates: 20g; Phosphorus: 280mg; Potassium: 189mg; Sodium: 25mg; Protein: 27g

HEALTHY HERBY TURKEY BURGERS

SERVES 2 / PREP TIME: 15 MINUTES / COOK TIME: 35 MINUTES

A delicious lunch or dinner.

---

5 OZ LEAN GROUND TURKEY MEAT	2 TBSP OLIVE OIL
1 WHITE ONION, FINELY DICED	PINCH OF BLACK PEPPER TO TASTE
1 CELERY STALK, FINELY DICED	2 HAMBURGER ROLLS
1 RED BELL PEPPER, FINELY DICED	1/2 CUP ARUGULA/BABY SPINACH
1 TSP DILL	
1 TSP CILANTRO	
1 TSP DRY MUSTARD	

---

1. Pre-heat oven to 400°F/200 °C/Gas Mark 6.
2. Mix the vegetables, olive oil, pepper and herbs in a medium bowl.
3. Add the meat to the vegetables and mix together until combined.
4. Use wet hands to 2 create burgers.
5. Place the burgers on a lightly oiled baking tray and bake in the oven for 25-30 minutes or until meat is cooked through (use a knife in the centre to check; the juices should run clear).
6. Serve in the hamburger roll and top with arugula/spinach and a helping of extra mustard as desired.

Top tip: an egg helps the burger mixture to stick so try adding 1 egg white before the meat, but remember to note how much protein you are consuming.

Per serving: Calories: 476; Fat: 22g; Carbohydrates: 30g; Phosphorus: 280mg; Potassium: 492mg; Sodium: 289mg; Protein: 24g

CHICKEN, GINGER & BEAN SPROUT STIR FRY

SERVES 2 / PREP TIME: 5 MINUTES / COOK TIME: 30 MINUTES

A Chinese influenced fresh stir fry dish.

---

1 TSP COCONUT OIL

1 CUP RICE NOODLES, UNSALTED

1X 3OZ SKINLESS CHICKEN BREAST

1/8 CUP CELERY, CHOPPED

1/4 CUP SCALLIONS, CHOPPED

1/4 CUP BEANSPROUTS

1 TSP FRESH GINGER, GRATED

1/2 GARLIC CLOVE, MINCED

1/2 LIME

---

1. Boil a pan of water on a high heat and add noodles. Cook for 10-15 minutes or according to package guidelines.
2. Meanwhile, heat oil in a wok on a high heat and add chopped chicken breasts, cooking for 15-20 minutes or until thoroughly cooked and place to one side.
3. Add celery and bean sprouts to the wok and cook for 10 minutes before adding scallions, ginger, garlic and cooked chicken back into the pan.
4. Stir through for a few minutes until piping hot throughout and add noodles to the wok after draining.
5. Serve with the juice of your lime squeezed over the top.

Per serving: Calories: 250; Fat: 11g; Carbohydrates: 30g; Phosphorus: 105mg; Potassium: 187mg; Sodium: 139mg; Protein: 12g

CHICKEN BREAST & CRANBERRIES

SERVES 2 / PREP TIME: 2 MINUTES / COOK TIME: 30 MINS

Juicy chicken served with red cabbage.

---

1 TSP EXTRA VIRGIN OLIVE OIL

1/8 RED ONION, FINELY SLICED

2X 3OZ SKINLESS, CHICKEN BREASTS

1/2 RED CABBAGE, SLICED AND SOAKED
IN WARM WATER

1 TSP NUTMEG

1 TSP APPLE VINEGAR

1/2 CUP CRANBERRIES

1 TSP BROWN SUGAR

---

1. Bring a pan of water to boiling point and add the sliced red cabbage with the nutmeg and cinnamon to the water.
2. Cover and simmer for 15-20 minutes.
3. Meanwhile, heat the oil in a skillet on a medium to high heat.
4. Add the onions and saute for 5-6 minutes until soft.
5. Now add the chicken breasts for 10 minutes on each side.
6. In a separate small pan, add the cranberries with water to cover and the apple vinegar and brown sugar.
7. Bring to a boil and then turn down heat and simmer for 10 minutes or until cranberries are soft. Keep an eye on water levels and top up if necessary.
8. Once the cranberries are soft, blend in a food processor until smooth.
9. Drain the cabbage and season with black pepper.
10. Serve chicken breast on a bed of red cabbage and drizzle cranberry sauce over to taste.

Per serving: Calories: 150; Fat: 10g; Carbohydrates: 7g; Phosphorus: 113mg; Potassium: 134mg; Sodium: 64 mg; Protein: 20g

MOROCCAN CHICKEN CURRY

SERVES 2 / PREP TIME: 10 MINUTES / COOK TIME: 35 MINUTES

Spicy turmeric and cumin with chicken and eggplant curry.

---

1 TBSP COCONUT OIL

1 TSP GARAM MASALA

1 TSP CUMIN

1 TSP TURMERIC

1/2 ONION, DICED

1 CLOVE GARLIC, MINCED

1 EGGPLANT, SOAKED IN WARM WATER AND CUBED

1/2 CUP CHOPPED TOMATOES, NO ADDED SALT OR SUGAR

1 CUP WATER

2X 3OZ SKINLESS CHICKEN/TURKEY BREASTS, CHOPPED

2 TBSP FRESH CILANTRO, FINELY CHOPPED

2 CUP BROWN RICE

---

1. Heat oil in a pan on a medium heat and add onions, stirring for 3-4 minutes until they begin to soften.
2. Add spices one by one and stir for 4-5 minutes, releasing the flavors.
3. Now add the garlic and stir.
4. Add the tomatoes and water to the pan and stir thoroughly.
5. Now add the chicken pieces and eggplant, cover and simmer for 25-30 minutes until chicken is completely cooked through.
6. Meanwhile prepare your rice by bringing a pan of water to the boil, adding rice-cover and simmer for 20 minutes.
7. Drain and cover the rice and return to the stove for 5 minutes.
8. Serve individual rice portions and the chicken curry over the top.
9. Sprinkle with fresh cilantro to serve.

Per serving: Calories: 204; Fat: 5g; Carbohydrates: 25g; Phosphorus: 113mg; Potassium: 250mg; Sodium: 50mg; Protein: 12g

CUMIN KEBABS WITH LIME & CILANTRO DIP

SERVES 2 / PREP TIME: 15 MINUTES / COOK TIME: 25 MINS

Middle Eastern inspired chicken kebabs.

FOR THE CHICKEN:

1/2 CUP LEMON JUICE

2 GARLIC CLOVES, MINCED

1 TSP THYME, FINELY CHOPPED

1 TSP PAPRIKA

1 TSP GROUND CUMIN

1/2 TSP CAYENNE PEPPER

2X 3OZ SKINLESS CHICKEN BREASTS, CUBED

2 METAL KEBAB SKEWERS

LEMON WEDGES TO GARNISH

FOR THE DIP:

1/2 RED ONION, FINELY DICED

1/2 RED BELL PEPPER, FINELY DICED

1 TSP EXTRA VIRGIN OLIVE OIL

1/2 LIME, JUICED

1 TSP BLACK PEPPER

1 TBSP FRESH CILANTRO, FINELY CHOPPED

---

1. Whisk the lemon juice, garlic, thyme, paprika, cumin, and cayenne pepper in a bowl.
2. Skewer the chicken cubes using kebab sticks (metal).
3. Baste the chicken on each side with the marinade, covering for as long as possible in the fridge (the lemon juice will tenderize the meat which is great for anti-inflammation, one of the symptoms of kidney disease).
4. When ready to cook, preheat the oven to 400°F/200 °C/Gas Mark 6 and bake for 20-25 minutes or until chicken is thoroughly cooked through.
5. Prepare the salsa by mixing all salsa ingredients in a separate bowl.
6. Serve the chicken kebabs, garnished with the lemon wedges and the salsa on the side.

Per serving: Calories: 156; Fat: 5g; Carbohydrates: 7g; Phosphorus: 150mg; Potassium: 384mg; Sodium: 58 mg; Protein: 20g

LOW FAT TURKEY AND ZUCCHINI PASTA

SERVES 2 / PREP TIME: 1 HOUR / COOK TIME: 30 MINUTES

Zucchini pasta is so delicious and pairs excellently with the turkey.

FOR THE TURKEY:

3OZ SKINLESS TURKEY BREAST, SLICED

1 TBSP EXTRA VIRGIN OLIVE OIL

JUICE OF 1/4 LEMON

1/2 CLOVE GARLIC, CRUSHED

1/2 TSP DRIED OREGANO

PINCH OF BLACK PEPPER

FOR THE PASTA:

1 1/2 LARGE ZUCCHINI,

1 TSP EXTRA VIRGIN OLIVE OIL

1. Marinate the turkey slices in 1 tbsp olive oil, lemon, garlic, oregano and pepper for at least 1 hour and up to overnight.
2. Pre-heat oven to 400°F/200°C/Gas Mark 6 when ready to cook.
3. Line a baking sheet with foil or parchment paper.
4. Layer the turkey strips on the baking tray and cook for 20-25 minutes or until cooked through.
5. Meanwhile, prepare your zucchini by slicing into thin spaghetti strips – use a mandolin or spiralyzer and leave in a colander to drain for 10 minutes.
6. When turkey is cooked through, remove from oven and place to one side.
7. Boil a pan of water on a medium heat and add a pinch of black pepper.
8. Add your zucchini spaghetti to the water and boil for 2 minutes before immediately draining.
9. Plate and serve, layering the turkey on top and drizzling with 1 tsp olive oil and a little black pepper.
10. Top tip: If you're in a rush this will still taste delicious without the marinating time, just coat your turkey and cook straight away.

Per serving: Calories: 180; Fat: 15g; Carbohydrates: 2g; Phosphorus: 75mg; Potassium: 197mg; Sodium: 196mg; Protein: 9g

NUTTY PESTO CHICKEN

SERVES 2 / PREP TIME: 10 MINUTES / COOK TIME: 35 MINUTES

An amazing chicken dish for the two of you!

2X 3OZ SKINLESS CHICKEN OR TURKEY BREASTS

1 BUNCH OF FRESH BASIL

1/2 CUP RAW SPINACH

1 CUP CRUSHED WALNUTS

2 TBSP EXTRA VIRGIN OLIVE OIL

1/4 CUP BRIE (OPTIONAL)

1/2 CUP ARUGULA

---

1. Preheat oven to 350°f/170°c/Gas Mark 4.
2. Take the chicken breasts and use a meat pounder to 'thin' each breast into 1cm thick escalopes.
3. Reserve a handful of the nuts and arugula.
4. Add the rest of the ingredients and a little black pepper to a blender or pestle and mortar and blend until smooth (you can leave this a little chunky for a rustic feel if you wish).
5. Add a little water if the pesto needs thinning.
6. Coat the chicken in the pesto.
7. Bake the chicken in the oven for at least 30 minutes or until chicken is completely cooked through.
8. Top each chicken escalope with the remaining nuts and place under the broiler for 5 minutes for a crispy topping to complete.
9. Serve on a bed of arugula.

Per serving: Calories: 360; Fat: 53g; Carbohydrates: 9g; Phosphorus: 350mg; Potassium: 511mg; Sodium: 119mg; Protein: 32g

HERBY TURKEY MEATBALLS

SERVES 2 / PREP TIME: 10 MINUTES / COOK TIME: 30 MINUTES

Succulent meatballs and spaghetti.

5 OZ LEAN TURKEY MINCE	FOR THE SAUCE:
2 GARLIC CLOVES, CRUSHED	1 TBSP EXTRA VIRGIN OLIVE OIL
1/4 CUP 100% WHITE BREADCRUMBS	1 RED ONION, FINELY CHOPPED
1 TBSP PARSLEY	1/2 CAN CHOPPED TOMATOES (NO ADDED SALT OR SUGAR)
1 TBSP EXTRA VIRGIN OLIVE OIL	1/2 CUP OF WATER
1 CUP SPAGHETTI	

1. Mix the turkey mince with garlic, breadcrumbs and herbs in a bowl.
2. Season with a little black pepper and separate into 8 balls using your hands.
3. Heat 1/2 tbsp oil in a pan over a medium heat and add onion, sautéing for a few minutes until softened.
4. Add the tomatoes and ½ cup water.
5. Cover and lower heat to simmer for 15 minutes.
6. Meanwhile, boil your water and cook spaghetti to recommended guidelines.
7. In a separate pan, heat 1/2 tbsp oil and add the meatballs, turning carefully to brown the surface of each.
8. Continue this for 5-7 minutes before adding the meatballs to the sauce and simmering for a further 10 minutes.
9. Drain spaghetti, portion up and pour a half the meatballs and sauce over the top to serve.

Per serving: Calories: 568; Fat: 20g; Carbohydrates: 34g; Phosphorus: 254mg; Potassium: 69mg ; Sodium: 42mg; Protein: 24g

MEATS (BEEF, PORK & LAMB)

PORK BURGERS WITH RED CABBAGE SLAW

SERVES 2 / PREP TIME: 15 MINUTES / COOK TIME: 3-4 HOURS

Sweet and Savory.

---

6 OZ BONELESS PORK SHOULDER ROAST

1 ONION, SLICED

3 CLOVES GARLIC

1 TBSP EXTRA VIRGIN OLIVE OIL

1 CUP WATER

3 TBSP RED WINE VINEGAR

1 TSP BLACK PEPPER

1/4 RED CABBAGE, SLICED

1 TSP CINNAMON

1 TSP NUTMEG

2 BUNS TO SERVE

---

1. Preheat oven to 350°f/180°c/Gas Mark 5.
2. Soak vegetables in warm water.
3. Meanwhile, cut the pork into cubes.
4. In a skillet, cook the pork, onions and garlic in oil over a medium heat for 5 minutes.
5. Add ingredients to a baking dish, along with the water, red wine vinegar and black pepper.
6. Cover and bake for 3-4 hours.
7. Remove the cover and continue to cook for 30 minutes.
8. Meanwhile, add the cabbage, nutmeg and cinnamon with water to cover into a pot over a high heat and bring to a boil.
9. Turn down the heat and allow to simmer for 15-20 minutes or until cabbage is soft.
10. Remove pork from the oven and allow to cool before shredding the meat with a fork.
11. Serve the pork meat in the buns with the red cabbage.
12. Enjoy!

Per serving: Calories: 323; Fat: 17g; Carbohydrates: 24g; Phosphorus: 323mg; Potassium: 137mg ; Sodium: 52mg; Protein: 25g

BEEF BURGERS & BRIE

SERVES 2 / PREP TIME: 10 MINUTES / COOK TIME: 20 MINUTES

Succulent beef burgers, oozing with brie cheese and mustard.

6OZ LEAN 100% GRASS-FED GROUND BEEF

1 TSP BLACK PEPPER

1 GARLIC CLOVE, MINCED

1 TSP COCONUT OIL

2 ONIONS, FINELY DICED

1 TBSP BALSAMIC VINEGAR

4 SLICES BRIE CHEESE

1 TSP MUSTARD

2 HAMBURGER ROLLS

1. Season ground beef with pepper and herbs and then mix in minced garlic.
2. Form burger shapes with the ground beef using the palms of your hands.
3. Heat a skillet on a medium to high heat, and then add the coconut oil.
4. Sauté the onions for 5-10 minutes until browned.
5. Then add in the balsamic vinegar and sauté for another 5 minutes.
6. Remove and set aside.
7. Add the burgers to the pan and heat on the same heat for 5-6 minutes before flipping and heating for a further 5-6 minutes until cooked through.
8. Add the brie slices to the top of each burger whilst still in the skillet.
9. Spread the mustard onto the burger rolls and top with the burger and brie.
10. Stuff with arugula or lettuce of your choice and serve right away!

Top tip: If using fresh beef and not defrosted, prepare double the ingredients and freeze burgers in plastic wrap (after cooling) for up to 1 month. Thoroughly defrost before heating through completely in the oven to serve.

Per serving: Calories: 358; Fat: 18g; Carbohydrates: 23g; Phosphorus: 216mg; Potassium: 511mg ; Sodium: 119 mg; Protein: 23g

THAI LAMB CURRY

SERVES 2 / PREP TIME: 10 MINUTES / COOK TIME: 45 MINUTES

Fresh, zingy and hot all at the same time!

---

5 OZ LAMB STEAK, SLICED INTO STRIPS

1 TBSP COCONUT OIL

1 GARLIC CLOVE, MINCED

1/2 STICK OF LEMON GRASS, VERY FINELY DICED

1/4 CUP OF HOMEMADE CHICKEN BROTH

1/4 CUP LOW FAT COCONUT MILK

1/2 TSP CURRY POWDER

1/2 ONION, CHOPPED

1 TBSP OF FRESH GINGER, GRATED

1/2 CUP OF TENDER-STEM OR SPROUTING BROCCOLI

1 STEM OF GREEN ONION, SLICED

1 CUPS COOKED BROWN RICE

---

1. Heat the coconut oil and garlic in a large pan over a medium to high heat for 2 minutes.
2. Add the lamb slices to the pan and brown each side for 2 minutes.
3. Once browned, remove lamb from the plan and place to one side.
4. Mix the ginger, curry powder, lemongrass and ¼ of the homemade chicken broth in a separate bowl.
5. Pour the broth mix, along with the broccoli into the pan.
6. Add the beef back into the pan along with the chopped onions.
7. Add the last of the broth and coconut milk over the lamb and simmer for 30-40 minutes or until piping hot and the beef is soft.
8. Serve piping hot with the green onion scattered over the top and rice on the side.

Per serving: Calories: 339; Fat: 17g; Carbohydrates: 35g; Phosphorus: 261mg; Potassium: 139mg ; Sodium: 15mg; Protein: 25g

SPICED LAMB BURGERS

SERVES 2 / PREP TIME: 10 MINUTES / COOK TIME: 20 MINUTES

Juicy burgers with a yogurt dip.

---

6 OZ LEAN GROUND LAMB

1/2 RED ONION, FINELY DICED

1 TSP HARISSA SPICES

1 TBSP PARSLEY

1 TBSP EXTRA VIRGIN OLIVE OIL

1 LEMON, JUICED

1 CLOVE OF GARLIC, MINCED

1/2 CUP OF LOW FAT PLAIN YOGURT TO SERVE (OPTIONAL)

1 TSP CUMIN

1 CUP ARUGULA

---

1. Preheat the broiler on a medium to high heat.
2. Mix together the ground lamb, red onion, parsley, Harissa spices and olive oil until combined.
3. Shape 1 inch thick patties using wet hands.
4. Add the patties to a baking tray and place under the broiler for 7-8 minutes on each side or until thoroughly cooked through.
5. Mix the yogurt, lemon juice and cumin and serve over the lamb burgers with a side salad of arugula.

Per serving: Calories: 306; Fat: 20g; Carbohydrates: 10g; Phosphorus: 269mg; Potassium: 492mg ; Sodium: 86mg; Protein: 23g

PORK LOINS WITH LEEKS

SERVES 2 / PREP TIME: 10 MINUTES / COOK TIME: 35 MINUTES

Delicious!

1 TBSP DRY MUSTARD	2X 3 OZ PORK TENDERLOIN
1 TBSP MUSTARD SEEDS	1 LEEK, SLICED
1 TBSP CUMIN SEEDS	1 TSP EXTRA VIRGIN OLIVE OIL

1. Preheat the broiler to a medium high heat.
2. In a dry skillet heat mustard and cumin seeds until they start to pop (3-5 minutes).
3. Grind seeds using a pestle and mortar or blender and then mix in the dry mustard.
4. Coat the pork on both sides with the mustard blend and add to a baking tray to broil for 25-30 minutes or until cooked through. Turn once half way through.
5. Remove and place to one side.
6. Heat the oil in a pan on a medium heat and add the leeks for 5-6minutes or until soft.
7. Serve the pork tenderloin on a bed of leeks and enjoy!

Per serving: Calories: 139; Fat: 5g; Carbohydrates: 2g; Phosphorus: 278mg; Potassium: 45mg ; Sodium: 47mg; Protein: 18g

CHINESE BEEF WRAPS

SERVES 2 / PREP TIME: 10 MINUTES / COOK TIME: 30 MINUTES

Fresh cucumber and lettuce with chinese beef.

1 GARLIC CLOVE, MINCED	1 TBSP RICE WINE VINEGAR
1/2 CUCUMBER, DICED	1 TSP GROUND GINGER
5 OZ LEAN GROUND BEEF	2 ICEBERG LETTUCE LEAVES
1 TBSP CHILI FLAKES	1 TSP CANOLA OIL

1. Mix the ground meat with the garlic, rice wine vinegar, chili flakes and ginger in a bowl.
2. Heat oil in a skillet over a medium heat.
3. Add the beef to the pan and cook for 20-25 minutes or until cooked through.
4. Serve beef mixture with diced cucumber in each lettuce wrap and fold.

Per serving: Calories: 156; Fat: 2g; Carbohydrates: 4; Phosphorus: 1mg; Potassium: 78mg ; Sodium: 54mg; Protein: 14g

LAMB MOUSSAKA

SERVES 2 / PREP TIME: 10 MINUTES / COOK TIME: 50 MINUTES

A Greek inspired dish.

---

1 GARLIC CLOVE, MINCED

1 ONION, DICED

6 OZ LEAN GROUND LAMB

1 TSP CAYENNE PEPPER

1 TSP PARSLEY

1/2 CUP WATER

1 TSP BLACK PEPPER

1 EGGPLANT, SLICED

FOR THE WHITE SAUCE:

1/4 CUP ALL PURPOSE WHITE FLOUR

3/4 CUP RICE MILK (UNENRICHED)

1 TBSP BUTTER

1/4 TEASPOON WHITE PEPPER

1 TSP BLACK PEPPER

---

1. Preheat the oven to 350°f/170°c/Gas Mark 4.
2. Soak vegetables in warm water.
3. To prepare white sauce: Heat saucepan on a medium heat.
4. Add the butter to the pan on the side nearest to the handle.
5. Tilt the pan towards you and allow butter to melt, whilst trying not to let it cover the rest of the pan.
6. Now add the flour to the opposite side of the pan and gradually mix the flour into the butter - continue to mix until smooth.
7. Add the milk and mix thoroughly for 10 minutes until lumps dissolve.
8. Add pepper.
9. Turn off the heat and place to one side.
10. To prepare the moussaka: Heat oil in a skillet on a medium to high heat and add onions and garlic for 5 minutes until soft.
11. Add lamb mince, season with herbs and spices, add water and cook for 10-15 minutes or until completely browned.
12. Layer an oven proof dish with 1/3 eggplant slices.
13. Add 1/3 beef mince on top.
14. Layer with 1/3 white sauce.
15. Repeat until ingredients are used.
16. Cover and add to the oven for 25-30 minutes or until golden and bubbly.
17. Remove and serve piping hot!

Per serving: Calories: 227; Fat: 7g; Carbohydrates: 23; Phosphorus: 278mg; Potassium: 183mg ; Sodium: 90mg; Protein: 18g

BEEF STROGANOFF

SERVES 2 / PREP TIME: 10 MINUTES / COOK TIME: 4-5 HOURS

Healthy and filling.

1/2 ONION, DICED

1 GARLIC CLOVE, MINCED

6 OZ LEAN FRYING BEEF

1 CUP HOMEMADE CHICKEN OR VEGETABLE STOCK

1 TSP DRIED OREGANO

1 TBSP BLACK PEPPER

1/2 CUP LOW FAT SOUR CREAM

1/4 CUP ALL-PURPOSE WHITE FLOUR

2 TBSP WATER

1 CUP BROWN RICE

---

1. Soak vegetables in warm water prior to cooking.
2. In a crockpot or slow cooker, add the pepper, oregano, garlic, onion, stock and beef.
3. Cover and cook on high for 4-5 hours or until beef is tender.
4. Add the water, flour and sour cream to the crock pot and mix until smooth.
5. Continue to cook for another 20 minutes or until the mixture has thickened.
6. Meanwhile, bring a pan of water to the boil and add the rice for 20 minutes.
7. Drain the water from the rice, add the lid and steam for 5 minutes.
8. Serve the rice with the creamy beef over the top and enjoy!

Per serving: Calories: 545; Fat: 24g; Carbohydrates: 48; Phosphorus: 260mg; Potassium: 199mg ; Sodium: 52mg; Protein: 30g

CRISPY CHILI BEEF & RICE

SERVES 2 / PREP TIME: 10 MINUTES / COOK TIME: 30 MINUTES

A tasty and filling dinner.

1 ONION, DICED	1 TSP CHILI POWDER
1 RED BELL PEPPER, DICED	1 TSP OREGANO
2 GARLIC CLOVES, MINCED	2 TBSP EXTRA VIRGIN OLIVE OIL
6 OZ LEAN GROUND BEEF	1 CUP WATER
	1 CUP WILD RICE
	1 TBSP FRESH CILANTRO TO SERVE

1. Soak vegetables in warm water prior to cooking.
2. Bring a pan of water to the boil and add rice for 20 minutes.
3. Meanwhile, add the oil to a pan and heat on a medium to high heat.
4. Add the onions, pepper and garlic and saute for 5 minutes until soft.
5. Remove and set aside.
6. Add the beef to the pan and stir until browned.
7. Add the vegetables back into the pan and stir.
8. Now add the chili powder and herbs and the water, cover and turn the heat down a little to simmer for 15 minutes.
9. Meanwhile, drain the water from the rice, add the lid and steam while the chili is cooking.
10. Serve beef and rice hot with the fresh cilantro sprinkled over the top.

Per serving: Calories: 459; Fat: 22g; Carbohydrates: 36; Phosphorus: 332mg; Potassium: 360mg ; Sodium: 33mg; Protein: 22g

MINTED LAMB WITH ROOT VEG

SERVES 2 / PREP TIME: 10 MINUTES / COOK TIME: 4-5 HOURS

A satisfying roast dish.

6OZ LEAN LAMB SHOULDER	1 TSP BLACK PEPPER
1 TBSP MINT, CHOPPED	2 TBSP EXTRA VIRGIN OLIVE OIL
1 TURNIP, CUBED	1 TSP THYME
1 RUTABAGA, CUBED	1 TSP ROSEMARY
	2 GARLIC CLOVES, CHOPPED

---

1. Preheat oven to its highest setting.
2. Soak the vegetables in warm water.
3. Trim any fat from the lamb shoulder.
4. Rub the lamb with 1tbsp olive oil, pepper and herbs.
5. Line a baking tray with the rest of the olive oil, turnip and rutabaga.
6. Add the lamb shoulder and cover with foil.
7. Turn the oven down to 325°f/170°c/Gas Mark 3 and add the dish into the oven.
8. Cook for 4-5 hours, remove and rest.
9. Slice the lamb with a carving knife and serve on a bed of the juicy roasted vegetables.

Per serving: Calories: 282; Fat: 19g; Carbohydrates: 12; Phosphorus: 310mg; Potassium: 344mg ; Sodium: 44mg; Protein: 24g

SEAFOOD

SEABASS WITH PESTO MASH

SERVES 2 / PREP TIME: 5 MINUTES / COOK TIME: 15 MINUTES

Great for the kidneys!

---

2 X 3OZ SEA BASS FILLETS

1 TSP BLACK PEPPER

1 TBSP EXTRA VIRGIN OLIVE OIL

FOR THE MASH:

2 TURNIPS, PEELED AND CUBED

FOR THE PESTO:

1/2 CUP FRESH BASIL

1/2 CUP FRESH SPINACH

1 TSP BLACK PEPPER

1/4 CUP EXTRA VIRGIN OLIVE OIL

1 GARLIC CLOVE, MINCED

1 LEMON, JUICED

---

1. Soak all your vegetables in warm water.
2. Prepare the pesto by blending all the ingredients for the pesto in a food processor or grinding with a pestle and mortar. Place to one side.
3. Boil a pan of water on a high heat and add the turnips.
4. Allow to boil for 20-25 minutes or until very soft.
5. Drain and use a potato masher to mash the turnips.
6. Fold the pesto through the mash.
7. Now grab a skillet and heat the oil over a medium to high heat.
8. Sprinkle black pepper over the sea bass fillet and score the skin of the fish a few times with a sharp knife.
9. Add the sea bass fillet to the very hot pan with the skin side down.
10. Cook for 7-8 minutes and turn over (this will allow the skin to turn crispy and golden).
11. Cook for a further 3-4 minutes or until cooked through.
12. Remove fillets from the skillet and allow to rest.

Per serving: Calories: 410; Fat: 35g; Carbohydrates: 5; Phosphorus: 261mg; Potassium: 236mg ; Sodium: 99mg; Protein: 17g

TILAPIA CEVICHE

SERVES 2 / PREP TIME: 2 HOURS / COOK TIME: 10 MINUTES

Enjoy for lunch or as a starter!

2X 3OZ FRESH TILAPIA FILLETS

1/2 RED ONION, FINELY DICED

1/2 RED BELL PEPPER, FINELY DICED

2 TBSP FRESH CILANTRO

1/4 CUP OLIVE OIL

1 TSP BLACK PEPPER

1 LIME

4 CRACKERS/SLICES OF MELBA TOAST

---

1. Preheat the broiler on a medium to high heat.
2. Cut tilapia into small bite size pieces.
3. Place tilapia under the broiler for 7-10 minutes or until cooked through.
4. Remove and allow to cool in a separate bowl, before squeezing the juice from the lime over the top and mixing well.
5. Mix the bell pepper, onion, cilantro, mango, pepper and oil with the cooked tilapia and marinate for a minimum of 2 hours in the refrigerator.
6. Divide into two and serve with crackers/toast for a tasty lunch or starter.

Per serving: Calories: 389; Fat: 29g; Carbohydrates: 18g; Phosphorus: 183mg; Potassium: 217mg ; Sodium: 134mg; Protein: 17g

SWEET & SOUR SWORDFISH

SERVES 2 / PREP TIME: 30 MINUTES / COOK TIME: 15 MINUTES

The meaty flavors combine deliciously with the fresh herbs and hot kick of the chili in this fish dish.

2X 3OZ SWORDFISH FILLETS	1 RED CHILI, FINELY DICED
4 TSP FRESH CILANTRO	1/4 CUP PINEAPPLE, CUBED
1 ONION, FINELY DICED	1 TBSP EXTRA VIRGIN OLIVE OIL
1 TSP BROWN SUGAR	1 GARLIC CLOVE, MINCED

1. Soak vegetables in warm water.
2. Meanwhile, add fish to an oven proof baking dish.
3. Whisk cilantro, onion, sugar, chili, lemon juice, oil and garlic in a separate bowl.
4. Add the pineapple chunks to the marinade.
5. Pour the marinade over the swordfish and turn fish over to coat both sides.
6. Cover and marinate in the refrigerator for at least 30 minutes.
7. Preheat the broiler to a medium heat when ready to cook.
8. Place oven dish under the broiler for 6-7 minutes on each side or until fish flakes easily with a fork.
9. Serve hot.

Per serving: Calories: 239; Fat: 10g; Carbohydrates: 11g; Phosphorus: 241mg; Potassium: 156mg ; Sodium: 100mg; Protein: 22g

MONKFISH PAELLA

SERVES 2 / PREP TIME: 10 MINUTES / COOK TIME: 35 MINUTES

Seasoned monkfish paella.

---

1 CUP BROWN RICE	2 TBSP EXTRA VIRGIN OLIVE OIL
3 CUPS OF WATER	1/4 TSP RED PEPPER FLAKES
6OZ MONKFISH FILLETS, DICED	1 TBSP PARSLEY, CRUSHED
2 GARLIC CLOVES, CRUSHED	1 LEMON, JUICE AND ZEST
1 WHITE ONION, DICED	1 LEMON – CUT INTO QUARTERS

---

1. Add the rice and 3 cups of water to a saucepan and boil on a high heat.
2. Once boiling, lower the heat, cover and simmer for 15 minutes.
3. Drain the rice and return to the heat for a further 3 minutes.
4. Place rice to one side.
5. In a skillet, heat the oil on a medium heat and then sauté the onion, garlic and red pepper flakes for 5 minutes until softened and then add the monkfish fillets.
6. Sauté for 6-9 minutes or until thoroughly cooked through and add the rice to the skillet.
7. Add in the parsley, zest and juice of 1 lemon, mixing well for a further 3-4 minutes.
8. Serve in a wide paella dish if possible or a large serving dish – scatter the lemon wedges around the edge and sprinkle with a little more fresh parsley.
9. Season with black pepper to taste.

Per serving: Calories: 335; Fat: 16g; Carbohydrates: 32g; Phosphorus: 262mg; Potassium: 188mg ; Sodium: 26mg; Protein: 15g

HONEY & LIME SALMON BURGERS

SERVES 2 / PREP TIME: 5 MINUTES / COOK TIME: 10 MINUTES

Healthy homemade version of the fast food favorite!

1/2 TSP HONEY

1/2 LIME, JUICED

1 BEATEN FREE RANGE EGG

5OZ CANNED WILD SALMON, DRAINED

2 SCALLIONS, CHOPPED

1 TBSP COCONUT OIL

2 TBSP FRESH GINGER, MINCED

---

1. Combine the salmon, egg, ginger, scallions and 1/2 tbsp oil in a bowl, mixing well with your hands to form 4 patties.
2. In a separate bowl, whisk the lime juice and honey until blended.
3. Heat 1/2 tbsp oil over a medium heat in a skillet and cook the patties for 4 minutes per side until firm and browned.
4. Glaze the top of each patty with the honey mixture and cook for another 15 seconds before you serve.
5. Serve with your favorite side salad or vegetables for a healthy treat.

Per serving: Calories: 291; Fat: 23g; Carbohydrates: 15g; Phosphorus: 310mg; Potassium: 74mg ; Sodium: 172mg; Protein: 15g

GARLIC, LEMON & PARSLEY HALIBUT

SERVES 2 / PREP TIME: 5 MINUTES / COOK TIME: 15 MINUTES

A meaty fish that tastes delicious with the citrus burst of the lemon.

1/2 LEMON

1 TBSP EXTRA VIRGIN OLIVE OIL

1 GARLIC CLOVE, MINCED

2X 3OZ HALIBUT STEAKS

2 TBSP UNSALTED BUTTER

2 TBSP WHITE ALL-PURPOSE FLOUR

1/2 CUP WATER

1 TBSP FRESH PARSLEY, FINELY CHOPPED

1 TSP BLACK PEPPER

---

1. Mix 1 tbsp lemon juice, garlic and olive oil in a large zip-lock bag, add the halibut fillets and allow to marinate for at least 5 minutes in the fridge.
2. Meanwhile, heat a non-stick skillet over a medium heat, before adding the halibut to the skillet and cooking for 5 minutes.
3. Turn the fish over before cooking for a further 4 minutes before moving and placing to one side.
4. To make the sauce, melt the butter in the skillet over a low heat.
5. Now add flour and stir.
6. Add in the flour and water and stir for 1 minute.
7. Mix in the black pepper, parsley and the rest of the lemon juice, stirring for 3 minutes until the sauce thickens.
8. Add the halibut back into the sauce and heat until piping hot throughout.
9. Serve with your favorite side salad or vegetables and enjoy.

Per serving: Calories: 306 ; Fat: 27g; Carbohydrates: 7g; Phosphorus: 238mg; Potassium: 30mg ; Sodium: 137mg; Protein: 9g

CHINESE STYLE SHRIMP

SERVES 2 / PREP TIME: 10 MINUTES / COOK TIME: 20 MINUTES

This sweet & sour shrimp is delicious.

1 CELERY STALK, FINELY DICED

3 GREEN ONIONS, FINELY DICED

1 RED BELL PEPPER, FINELY DICED

1/2 CUP CANNED, SLICED WATER CHESTNUTS (NO ADDED SALT OR SUGAR)

8 WHOLE SHRIMPS

1 TBSP CANOLA OIL

FOR THE SWEET AND SOUR SAUCE:

1 TBSP RED CHILI FLAKES

2 TBSP LEMON JUICE

1/2 CUP PINEAPPLE, FINELY DICED

1/3 CUP WATER

1 TBSP FRESH GINGER, GRATED

1. Soak vegetables in warm water.
2. Meanwhile, prepare shrimp by slicing down the middle (not all the way through) and pulling apart to 'butterfly' - leave heads and tails on.
3. Heat the oil in a skillet on a medium to high heat.
4. Add the chestnuts, peppers, onion and celery and saute for 5 minutes.
5. Remove vegetables and place to one side.
6. Combine the sweet and sour sauce ingredients in a separate bowl.
7. Pour over your shrimp on a baking tray and allow to marinate for as long as possible.
8. Preheat the broiler to a medium heat.
9. Add the shrimp under the broiler and broil for 12-15 minutes or until cooked through.
10. Serve shrimp with the vegetables and enjoy.

Per serving: Calories: 212; Fat: 10g; Carbohydrates: 23g; Phosphorus: 132mg; Potassium: 550mg ; Sodium: 260mg; Protein: 13g

TUNA SUPER SALAD

SERVES 2 / PREP TIME: 5 MINUTES / COOK TIME: 35 MINUTES

Fennel and lemon tuna salad.

5OZ TUNA IN SPRING WATER

2 TBSP OLIVE OIL

1 TSP CRUSHED BLACK PEPPERCORNS

1 TSP CRUSHED FENNEL SEEDS,

1/2 CUP FENNEL BULB, TRIMMED

1/2 CUP WATER

1 LEMON, JUICED

1 TSP FRESH PARSLEY, CHOPPED

1 CUP COOKED BROWN RICE

1 CUP FRESH GREEN BEANS, STEAMED

---

1. Mix tuna with oil, peppercorns and fennel seeds and rest for 10 minutes.
2. Heat the oil on a medium heat and sauté the fennel bulb slices for 5-6 minutes or until light brown.
3. Add the water to the pan and cook for 10 minutes until fennel is tender.
4. Stir in the lemon juice and lower heat to a simmer for another 5 minutes until liquid reduces.
5. Remove the fennel from the pan and slice.
6. Into an ovenproof dish add tuna mix with sliced fennel layered over the top and place under a broiler on a medium to high heat.
7. Broil for 5-6 minutes until top is crispy and brown.
8. Serve with brown rice, green beans on the side and parsley sprinkled over to garnish.

Per serving: Calories: 337 ; Fat: 16g; Carbohydrates: 34g; Phosphorus: 219mg; Potassium: 402mg ; Sodium: 263mg; Protein: 19g

CHILI & HONEY SEARED SALMON

SERVES 2 / PREP TIME: 15 MINUTES / COOK TIME: 15 MINUTES

Meaty fish served on a bed of salad.

2X 3OZ SKINLESS SALMON FILLETS

2 TBSP EXTRA VIRGIN OLIVE OIL

1 TBSP HONEY

1 TSP CHILI POWDER

1/2 FRESH LIME, JUICED

A PINCH OF BLACK PEPPER TO TASTE

FOR THE SALAD:

1 CUPS BABY ARUGULA LEAVES

1/2 CUP SLIVERED RED ONION

1 TBSP OLIVE OIL

1 TBSP BALSAMIC VINEGAR

---

1. In a bowl, marinate the salmon with 1 tbsp olive oil, lime juice, chili, honey and pepper and leave for at least 15 minutes (up to an hour).
2. Heat 1 tbsp oil in a skillet over a medium heat and cook the salmon skin-side down for 6-7 minutes on each side or until thoroughly cooked through.
3. Toss the arugula and onions with oil and vinegar in a separate bowl.
4. Serve the salmon fillets on the bed of salad.

Per serving: Calories: 334 ; Fat: 22g; Carbohydrates: 22g; Phosphorus: 229mg; Potassium: 499mg ; Sodium: 293mg; Protein: 17g

OVEN BAKED SPICED TROUT

SERVES 2 / PREP TIME: 5 MINUTES / COOK TIME: 15 MINUTES

Brilliantly baked trout fillets - perfect for lunch or dinner!

---

2 x 3OZ TROUT FILLETS	1 TSP CURRY POWDER
1 TBSP OLIVE OIL	1 TSP CAYENNE PEPPER
1/2 TSP PAPRIKA	1 LEMON, HALVED

---

1. Preheat oven to 350° F/180°c/Gas Mark 4.
2. Whisk together the oil and spices in a small bowl.
3. Wash and pat dry the trout fillets before coating both sides with oil and spices.
4. Add to a shallow baking dish with the lemon halves and garlic clove.
5. Bake uncovered for 20 to 30 minutes or until the trout fillets are thoroughly cooked through and flaky.
6. Serve with your choice of salad for a delicious summer time supper!

Per serving: Calories: 200; Fat: 13g; Carbohydrates: 3g; Phosphorus: 281mg; Potassium: 378mg ; Sodium: 45mg; Protein: 16g

VEGETARIAN

MEDITERRANEAN VEGETABLE LASAGNE

SERVES 2 / PREP TIME: 10 MINUTES / COOK TIME: 1 HOUR

Eggplant, zucchini and pepper.

1/2 CAN CHOPPED TOMATOES (NO ADDED SUGAR OR SALT)

1/2 CUP BABY SPINACH

1 TBSP EXTRA VIRGIN OLIVE OIL

1 GARLIC CLOVE, CRUSHED

2 TBSP OREGANO, DRIED

1/2 RED ONION, DICED

A PINCH OF BLACK PEPPER TO TASTE

1 ZUCCHINI , SLICED

1 RED BELL PEPPER, SLICED

1 EGGPLANT, SLICED

---

1. Preheat oven to 325°F/170 °C/Gas Mark 3 and soak vegetables in warm water prior to cooking.
2. Heat the olive oil in a skillet over a medium to high heat and add garlic and onions, sautéing for 4-5 minutes until soft.
3. Add the chopped tomatoes to the pan with the oregano and turn down to a simmer for 5 minutes.
4. Add the spinach to the sauce for 3-4 minutes until wilted and stir.
5. Layer the bottom of an oven/lasagne dish with 1/3 the eggplant slices and 1/3 red pepper slices and 1/3 zucchini slices.
6. Pour over 1/3 tomato sauce.
7. Repeat for a second layer.
8. Repeat for a third layer.
9. Bake in the oven for 45-50 minutes or until the vegetables are soft through to the centre (use your knife to test the middle).
10. Finish under the broiler until golden and bubbly.
11. Divide into portions and serve with a sprinkle of black pepper to taste.

Per serving: Calories: 125; Fat: 7g; Carbohydrates: 12g; Phosphorus: 87mg; Potassium: 460mg ; Sodium: 55mg; Protein: 2g

SPICY LIME TEMPAH BURGERS

SERVES 2 / PREP TIME: 5 MINUTES / COOK TIME: 15 MINUTES

These are wonderful in the summer and all year round for that matter!

EXTRA FIRM TEMPAH (2 PACKS)	1 CUCUMBER, FINELY DICED
2 TSP DRIED OREGANO	1 RED ONION, FINELY DICED
1/2 RED CHILI, FINELY DICED	1 CUP BABY SPINACH
1 LIME, JUICED	2 TBSP EXTRA VIRGIN OLIVE OIL
1 RED BELL PEPPER, DICED (OPTIONAL)	2 BUNS (OPTIONAL)

1. Marinate the tempah in 1 tbsp oil and oregano combined.
2. Soak vegetables in warm water and heat the broiler on a medium to high heat.
3. Prepare your cucumber salsa by mixing the cucumber with the red chili and lime juice.
4. Heat 1 tbsp extra olive oil in a skillet on a medium heat.
5. Sauté the onion in the skillet for 6-7 minutes or until caramelized.
6. Stir in the pepper and baby spinach for a further 3-4 minutes.
7. Place to one side.
8. Broil the tempah on a lined oven-proof dish for 4 minutes on each side.
9. Add the tempah to the bun and top with caramelized onion, spinach and diced peppers.
10. Serve immediately while hot with the cucumber salsa.

Per serving: Calories: 161; Fat: 8g; Carbohydrates: 0g; Phosphorus: 227mg; Potassium: 385mg ; Sodium: 169mg; Protein: 21g

MEXICAN PEPPER STEW

SERVES 2 / PREP TIME: 10 MINUTES / COOK TIME: 40 MINUTES

A Mexican inspired dish.

---

1 TBSP EXTRA VIRGIN OLIVE OIL	1 TSP BLACK PEPPER
1 ONION, CHOPPED	1 TSP CHILI FLAKES
1 YELLOW BELL PEPPER	1 TSP OREGANO, FRESH OR DRIED
1 GREEN BELL PEPPER, CHOPPED	1/2 CUP WATER
1 RED BELL PEPPER, CHOPPED	1 CUP RICE

---

1. Soak the vegetables in warm water prior to cooking.
2. Add the rice to a pan of water on a medium to high heat and cook for 20 minutes.
3. Meanwhile, heat the oil in a pot over a medium to high heat and add the onion for 5 minutes.
4. Season with herbs and spices before adding in peppers and stirring for 5 minutes.
5. Add water, cover and simmer for 25-30 minutes.
6. When the rice has soaked up most of the water, drain and replace the lid for 5 minutes with the heat on low.
7. Serve the pepper casserole with the rice on the side.

Per serving: Calories: 247; Fat: 9g; Carbohydrates: 39g; Phosphorus: 85mg; Potassium: 561mg ; Sodium: 15mg; Protein: 6g

GRILLED VEGETABLE FRITTATA

SERVES 2 / PREP TIME: 5 MINUTES / COOK TIME: 25 MINUTES

Delicious with a side of seasonal greens.

---

1 TBSP COCONUT OIL

1 CUP SWEETCORN

6 EGGS

1 CUP COCONUT MILK

1 TSP BLACK PEPPER

---

1. Preheat the broiler to a medium heat.
2. Whisk the eggs and coconut milk in a separate bowl.
3. On a medium heat, heat the coconut oil in an oven proof (steel) frying pan, adding in the corn and sautéing for 5 minutes.
4. Add the egg mix to the pan with the vegetables in and continue to cook on the stove (low heat) for 7 minutes until it becomes light and bubbly.
5. Finish the frittata in its pan under the broiler for a further 5 -10 minutes or until crispy on the top and cooked through.
6. Slice and serve hot or allow to cool and serve chilled from the fridge!

Per serving: Calories: 79; Fat: 6g; Carbohydrates: 3g; Phosphorus: 97mg; Potassium: 60mg ; Sodium: 59mg; Protein: 5g

ZUCCHINI, PEPPER & APRICOT TAGINE

SERVES 2 / PREP TIME: 5 MINUTES / COOK TIME: 35 MINUTES

A vegetarian take on the Moroccan classic.

---

2 TBSP COCONUT OIL

1 ONION, DICED

1 TURNIP, PEELED AND DICED

2 CLOVES OF GARLIC

1 TSP GROUND CUMIN

1/2 TSP GROUND GINGER

1/2 TSP GROUND CINNAMON

1/4 TSP CAYENNE PEPPER

1 ZUCCHINI, PEELED AND DICED

1 RED BELL PEPPER, DICED

1 CUP HOMEMADE VEGETABLE STOCK

2 TBSP LEMON JUICE

1/4 CUP CILANTRO, ROUGHLY CHOPPED

1/2 CAN APRICOTS, JUICES DRAINED

---

1. Soak the vegetables in warm water.
2. In a large pot, heat the oil on a medium high heat before sautéing the onion for 4-5 minutes until soft.
3. Add the turnip and cook for 10 minutes or until golden brown.
4. Add the garlic, cumin, ginger, cinnamon, and cayenne pepper, cooking for a further 3 minutes.
5. Add the carrots, red pepper, apricots and stock to the pot and then bring to the boil.
6. Turn the heat down to a medium heat, cover and simmer for 20 minutes.
7. Add the lemon juice towards the end of cooking.
8. Garnish with the cilantro.
9. Top tip: you can add potatoes or sweet potatoes to this dish, simply boil twice prior to cooking to lower the potassium.

Per serving: Calories: 196 ; Fat: 10g; Carbohydrates: 33g; Phosphorus: 116mg; Potassium: 542mg ; Sodium: 215mg; Protein: 3g

BASIL & GARLIC PASTA

SERVES 2 / PREP TIME: 5 MINUTES / COOK TIME: 20 MINUTES

Fresh and simple to make.

1/4 CUP FRESH BASIL, WASHED

1/4 CUP FRESH SPINACH/ARUGULA, WASHED

1 TSP BLACK PEPPER

1/8 CUP EXTRA VIRGIN OLIVE OIL

1/8 CUP OF WILD GARLIC LEAVES (2 GARLIC CLOVES AS ALTERNATIVE)

1/2 LEMON, JUICED

1 CUP FRESH GREEN BEANS, TRIMMED AND SOAKED IN WARM WATER

1 CUP FRESH WHITE PENNE PASTA

---

1. Bring a pan of water to the boil and add pasta, cooking for 15-20 minutes or according to package directions.
2. Meanwhile, blend all ingredients (minus green beans) in a food processor or a blender to reach required texture - chunky for a rustic feel or smooth as a dressing.
3. Add the green beans to steam over the pot of pasta for the last 10 minutes.
4. Drain pasta and stir through the pesto and green beans.
5. Serve with a sprinkle of black pepper to taste!

Per serving: Calories: 303; Fat: 14g; Carbohydrates: 16g; Phosphorus: 77mg; Potassium: 227mg ; Sodium: 71mg; Protein: 3g

BEAN SPROUT & TOFU STIR FRY

SERVES 2 / PREP TIME: 10 MINUTES / COOK TIME: 20 MINUTES

Easy yet scrumptious mid-week meal.

1/2 CUP SOFT TOFU

1 GARLIC CLOVE, MINCED

1 TBSP FRESH LIME JUICE

1 TBSP CANOLA OIL

1 CUP FRESH BROCCOLI FLORETS

1 TSP BLACK PEPPER

1/4 CUP BEAN SPROUTS

1 CUP COOKED BROWN RICE

---

1. Cut the tofu into cubes and soak the vegetables in warm water.
2. Heat a skillet on a medium to high heat and add the oil.
3. Once hot, add the tofu to the skillet and cook for 7-8 minutes or until golden brown.
4. Add the bean sprouts and broccoli and sauté for 7-8 minutes or until crisp.
5. Add the fresh lime juice.
6. Serve over rice and enjoy.

Per serving: Calories: 293; Fat: 12g; Carbohydrates: 25g; Phosphorus: 170mg; Potassium: 150mg ; Sodium: 140mg; Protein: 15g

ZUCCHINI SPAGHETTI

SERVES 2 / PREP TIME: 10 MINUTES / COOK TIME: 40 MINUTES

Gloriously healthy homemade pasta with a crunchy topping.

---

4 TURNIPS, PEELED AND CUT INTO FINE SHAVINGS

4 ZUCCHINIS, PEELED AND SLICED VERTICALLY TO MAKE NOODLES (USE A SPIRALIZER)

1 TSP CLEAR HONEY

1 TSP RED CHILI FLAKES

1 TBSP EXTRA VIRGIN OLIVE OIL

1/2 CUP ARUGULA

1/2 LEMON

---

1. Preheat the oven to 350°f/170°c/Gas Mark 4.
2. Soak the vegetables in warm water prior to cooking.
3. Spread the turnip slices over a baking tray and drizzle over honey before sprinkling with chili flakes.
4. Toss to coat.
5. Add to the oven for 35-40 minutes or until cooked through and slightly crispy.
6. Meanwhile, heat a pan of water on a high heat and bring to the boil.
7. Add the zucchini noodles and turn the heat down to simmer for 3-4 minutes.
8. Remove from the heat and place in a bowl of cold water immediately.
9. Serve zucchini noodles with turnip shavings and a drizzle of olive oil on top.
10. Mix the arugula with the lemon juice and serve on the side.
11. Enjoy!

Per serving: Calories: 187 ; Fat: 7g; Carbohydrates: 27g; Phosphorus: 258mg; Potassium: 435mg ; Sodium: 167mg; Protein: 6g

SPICED SQUASH STEW

SERVES 4 / PREP TIME: 10 MINUTES / COOK TIME: 40 MINUTES

A hearty, chunky dish packed full with flavor.

---

1 TBSP EXTRA VIRGIN OLIVE OIL

1 ONION, DICED

1 GARLIC CLOVE, CHOPPED

1/2 STALK CELERY, CHOPPED

1 TSP BLACK PEPPER

1 TSP TURMERIC

1 TSP CUMIN

1 TSP GINGER, GRATED

1/2 CAN CHOPPED TOMATOES (NO ADDED SALT OR SUGAR)

2 TBSP FRESH CILANTRO

1 CUP SPAGHETTI SQUASH

1 CUP WATER

---

1. In a large pot, heat the oil over a medium to high heat.
2. After 5 minutes, turn the heat down and sprinkle with spices and ginger.
3. Now add garlic and celery and continue to saute for 5 minutes.
4. Add the tomatoes and water along with half the cilantro and simmer.
5. Meanwhile prepare the squash by peeling and chopping into cubes.
6. Add the squash to the pan and continue to cook for 30 minutes, stirring occasionally.
7. Scatter with the rest of the cilantro to serve.

Per serving: Calories: 324; Fat: 19g; Carbohydrates: 44g; Phosphorus: 100mg; Potassium: 546mg ; Sodium: 185mg; Protein: 6g

RADISH, CHIVE & ASPARAGUS PIZZETTE

SERVES 2 / PREP TIME: 10 MINUTES / COOK TIME: 50 MINUTES

Healthy kidney pizza!

1/4 CUP OF CANNED CHOPPED TOMATOES (NO ADDED SALT OR SUGAR)

4 EGG WHITES

2 CRUSHED GARLIC CLOVES

1/4 CUP FRESH CHOPPED CHIVES

1 1/2 TBSP EXTRA VIRGIN OLIVE OIL

1/8 CUP BRIE

5 RADISHES, SLICED

1/4 CUP ASPARAGUS STEMS

---

1. Preheat oven to 350°f/180°c/Gas Mark 4.
2. Whisk the eggs and chives in a bowl and mix in the tomatoes.
3. Layer radishes, asparagus, garlic and onion slices in a round baking dish and drizzle with olive oil.
4. Roast in the oven for 15 minutes.
5. Pour the tomato and egg mixture over the vegetables in the baking dish.
6. Bake in the oven for 35-40 minutes, or until the centre is cooked through (check with a knife).
7. Sprinkle crumbled brie over the top and place under the broiler to brown.
8. Enjoy warm or cooled in the fridge with your favorite side salad.

Per serving: Calories: 177; Fat: 12g; Carbohydrates: 5g; Phosphorus: 161mg; Potassium: 153mg ; Sodium: 124mg; Protein: 10g

SIDES, SALADS AND SOUPS

SAVOURY PANCAKES

SERVES 2 / PREP TIME: 5 MINUTES / COOK TIME: 6 MINUTES

A great go-to made with your pantry essentials.

---

1 CUP OF CANNED PUMPKIN, NO ADDED SALT OR SUGAR

2 TBSP WATER

3 EGG WHITES

1 TBSP COCONUT OIL

1 TSP PAPRIKA

1 TSP CAYENNE PEPPER

1 TSP CINNAMON

---

1. Blend the pumpkin flesh together with water to form a smooth pulp.
2. Now add the rest of the ingredients (minus the coconut oil) and mix well.
3. Heat a large pan with coconut oil.
4. Pour the pumpkin mixture into the pan into individual rounded pancakes (go easy at first and pour your mixture into little circles, keep pouring whilst tilting the pan until you have a pancake to your desired shape).
5. Lift the mixture with a spatula and then flip. Cook for 3 minutes on either side.
6. Serve warm - they taste great with sweet or savory accompaniments.

Per serving: Calories: 136; Fat: 8g; Carbohydrates: 13g; Phosphorus: 63mg; Potassium: 377mg ; Sodium: 90mg; Protein: 7g

LIME & CARROT COLESLAW

SERVES 2 / PREP TIME: 15 MINUTES / COOK TIME: 0 MINUTES

Lovely healthy side dish or snack.

---

1 CARROT, PEELED AND FINELY SLICED

1 CUP WHITE CABBAGE, PEELED AND FINELY SLICED

1 LIME, JUICE AND ZEST

1 TBSP FRESH PARSLEY, FINELY CHOPPED

1 TBSP EXTRA VIRGIN OLIVE OIL

---

1. Soak vegetables in warm water for 5-10 minutes.
2. Drain and rinse with cold water.
3. Combine with the rest of the ingredients, cover and cool in refridgerator before serving.

Per serving: Calories: 314 ; Fat: 7g; Carbohydrates: 7g; Phosphorus: 18mg; Potassium: 220mg ; Sodium: 43mg; Protein: 1g

HOMEMADE RUTABAGA CHIPS

SERVES 2 / PREP TIME: 5 MINUTES / COOK TIME: 50 MINUTES

A healthy kidney friendly snack.

---

1 CUP RUTABAGA, PEELED AND SLICED

1 TBSP EXTRA VIRGIN OLIVE OIL

1 CHOPPED ONION

1 CLOVE MINCED GARLIC

1 TSP BLACK PEPPER

1 TSP OREGANO

1 TSP PAPRIKA

---

1. Heat oven to 375°f/190°c/Gas Mark 5.
2. Grease a baking tray with the olive oil.
3. Add turnip slices in a thin layer.
4. Dust over herbs and spices with an extra drizzle of olive oil.
5. Bake for 40-50 minutes (turning half way through to ensure even crispiness!)

Per serving: Calories: 150; Fat: 11g; Carbohydrates: 13g; Phosphorus: 62mg; Potassium: 386mg ; Sodium: 15mg; Protein: 2g

SPICY CABBAGE SOUP

SERVES 2 / PREP TIME: 10 MINUTES / COOK TIME: 35 MINUTES

A real zingy soup – great for winter but can be served cooled in the summer

---

2 TBSP OLIVE OIL

1 TSP MUSTARD SEEDS, GROUND

1 TSP CILANTRO SEEDS, GROUND

1 TSP CURRY POWDER

1 TBSP GINGER, MINCED

2 CUPS CABBAGE, THINLY SLICED

1 ONION, CHOPPED

ZEST AND JUICE OF 1 LIME

1 CUP LOW-SALT VEGETABLE BROTH OR HOMEMADE CHICKEN STOCK

BLACK PEPPER TO TASTE

3 CUPS OF WATER

---

1. In a pan on a medium heat, heat the oil then add the seeds and curry powder for 1 minute.
2. Add the ginger and cook for a further minute.
3. Then add in the cabbage, onions and the lime juice, cooking for at least 2 minutes or until the vegetables are soft.
4. Add the broth and allow to boil before turning the heat down slightly and simmering for 30 minutes.
5. Allow to cool.
6. Put the mixture in a food processor and puree until smooth.
7. Serve with lime zest and black pepper.

Per serving: Calories: 279 ; Fat: 19g; Carbohydrates: 28g; Phosphorus: 18mg; Potassium: 551mg ; Sodium: 232mg; Protein: 6g

ONION & TOMATO SOUP

SERVES 2 / PREP TIME: 10 MINUTES / COOK TIME: 45 MINUTES

Winter warming soup.

---

2 RED ONIONS

2 CUPS HOMEMADE CHICKEN STOCK

1 TBSP CANOLA OIL

1/2 CUP CANNED TOMATOES, NO ADD-ED SALT OR SUGAR

2 LARGE GARLIC CLOVES, CHOPPED

1 SPRIG OF THYME/1 TBSP DRIED THYME

1 TSP CHILI POWDER

---

1. Soak vegetables in warm water.
2. Heat oil in a large pan on a medium high heat before sweating the onions and garlic for 3-4 minutes.
3. Add the stock and canned tomatoes and bring to a boil over a high heat.
4. Turn down heat and allow to simmer for 25-30 minutes.
5. Now add the rest of the ingredients and simmer for a further 15 minutes or until the vegetables are tender.
6. Allow to cool slightly before blending in a food processor.
7. Add back to the pan on a medium heat and serve hot!

Per serving: Calories: 190; Fat: 15g; Carbohydrates: 15g; Phosphorus: 105mg; Potassium: 245mg ; Sodium: 111mg; Protein: 12g

GARLIC & PEPPER SOUP

SERVES 2 / PREP TIME: 10 MINUTES / COOK TIME: 45 MINUTES

Wonderfully satisfying!

---

4 RED BELL PEPPERS, CHOPPED

1/2 RED ONION, CHOPPED

1 GARLIC CLOVE, CHOPPED

1 1/2 CUPS HOMEMADE CHICKEN BROTH

1 HABANERO CHILI WITH THE STEMS REMOVED AND CHOPPED

1 TBSP OF EXTRA VIRGIN OLIVE OIL

---

1. In a pan on a medium heat, heat the oil then add the onions and peppers, sweating for 5 minutes.
2. Add the garlic cloves and chilis and saute for 3-4 minutes.
3. Add the broth and allow to boil before turning heat down slightly and simmering for 30 minutes.
4. Allow to cool.
5. Put the mixture in a food processor and puree until smooth.
6. Serve with lime zest and black pepper.

Per serving: Calories: 313 ; Fat: 20g; Carbohydrates: 16g; Phosphorus: 123mg; Potassium: 296mg ; Sodium: 71mg; Protein: 17g

VEGGIE COUSCOUS WITH APRICOTS

SERVES 2 / PREP TIME: 5 MINUTES / COOK TIME: NA

A great side dish for meats, fish or extra salad!

1/2 CUP DRY COUSCOUS

1/4 RED ONION, FINELY DICED

3 TBSP FRESH PARSLEY

1/4 CUP CANNED APRICOTS, JUICES DRAINED

1/4 EXTRA VIRGIN CUP OLIVE OIL

2 LEMONS

1 TSP BLACK PEPPER

---

1. Soak the vegetables in warm water.
2. Pour 1/2 cup boiling water over the couscous, cover and leave to sit for 5 minutes.
3. Drain any excess liquid from the couscous.
4. Drain the vegetables and add to the couscous, mixing well.
5. Add olive oil, lemon juice, herbs, apricots and pepper to the couscous mixture.
6. Serve straight away or refrigerate in an airtight container for 2-3 days.

Per serving: Calories: 355; Fat: 27g; Carbohydrates: 28g; Phosphorus: 43mg; Potassium: 257mg ; Sodium: 7mg; Protein: 3g

THAI BROTH

SERVES 2 / PREP TIME: 5 MINUTES / COOK TIME: 20 MINUTES

Fresh and full of delicious Asian-infused flavors.

---

1 TBSP OLIVE OIL

1/2 TBSP CILANTRO SEEDS

1/2 EGGPLANT, DICED

1/2 FRESH LIME

1/2 GARLIC CLOVE, MINCED

1 TSP MINCED GINGER

1/2 WHITE ONION, CHOPPED

1/4 CUP BABY SPINACH LEAVES

2 TBSP FRESH BASIL LEAVES

1/4 CUP OF HOMEMADE CHICKEN BROTH

1/4 CUP OF COCONUT MILK

1/2 RED CHILI, FINELY CHOPPED

1 STEM OF GREEN ONION, CHOPPED

---

1. Crush the fresh herbs and spices in a blender or pestle and mortar.
2. Mix in 1 tbsp of olive oil until a paste is formed.
3. Heat a large pan/wok with 1 tbsp olive oil on a high heat.
4. Fry the onions, garlic and ginger until soft but not crispy or browned.
5. Into the pan, add the spice paste from earlier along with the coconut milk and stir.
6. Slowly add the stock until a broth is formed.
7. Now add the eggplant and allow to simmer in the broth for 10-15 minutes.
8. Add the basil and spinach 2-3 minutes before the end of the cooking time.
9. Serve hot with the chili and green onion sprinkled over the top.

Per serving: Calories: 111 ; Fat: 6g; Carbohydrates: 10g; Phosphorus: 66mg; Potassium: 308mg ; Sodium: 202mg; Protein: 2g

TARRAGON & ROOT VEGETABLE MASH

SERVES 2 / PREP TIME: 5 MINUTES / COOK TIME:25 MINUTES

Try this home comfort with a little twist!

---

1 CUP RUTABAGA, PEELED AND CHOPPED

4 TURNIPS, PEELED AND CHOPPED

2 TBSP TARRAGON, FINELY CHOPPED

1 TBSP EXTRA VIRGIN OLIVE OIL

A PINCH OF BLACK PEPPER

---

1. Soak vegetables in warm water for 10 minutes.
2. Add the rutabaga and turnip to a large pan of water, bring to the boil, and cook for 15-20 minutes until vegetables very soft.
3. Drain and add the tarragon and olive oil to the vegetables and season with pepper.
4. Mash in a separate bowl using a potato masher or fork.
5. Serve hot! .

Per serving: Calories: 121; Fat: 7g; Carbohydrates: 15g; Phosphorus: 294mg; Potassium: 469mg ; Sodium: 135mg; Protein: 2g

CAULIFLOWER COUSCOUS

SERVES 2 / PREP TIME: 5 MINUTES / COOK TIME: 20 MINUTES

Spicy and delicious side dish.

---

2 TBSP EXTRA VIRGIN OLIVE OIL

1/4 CAULIFLOWER

1 LEMON, JUICE & ZEST

1 TSP CURRY POWDER

1/4 RED ONION, FINELY DICED

---

1. Soak vegetables in warm water prior to use.
2. Grate the cauliflower with a cheese grater.
3. In a large bowl, add cauliflower, red onion, lemon juice and curry powder.
4. Use your hands to toss the mixture and top with a little lemon zest to serve.
5. Refrigerate before serving or eat up straight away!

Per serving: Calories: 180; Fat: 14g; Carbohydrates: 13g; Phosphorus: 43mg; Potassium: 378mg ; Sodium: 27mg; Protein: 3g

STOCKS AND SAUCES

HOMEMADE TURKEY GRAVY

SERVES 2 / PREP TIME: 5 MINUTES / COOK TIME: 25 MINUTES

Kidney friendly gravy - just remember to add to your daily nutrient calculations.

3 OZ LEAN GROUND TURKEY, MINCED	1 TBSP CORNSTARCH
1 TSP GROUND SAGE	2 CUPS WATER
1 TSP GROUND BASIL	
1 TSP BLACK PEPPER	
1 TSP FENNEL SEEDS	

1. Combine the herbs and spices with the minced turkey.
2. Add a pot to the stove on a medium to high heat and cook the pork mix for 15 minutes or until cooked through.
3. Add the water and cornstarch to the pot and turn the heat down to simmer for a further 10 minutes.
4. Blend in a food processor until liquid consistency is reached and strain to get rid of any lumps.
5. Seal in an airtight container once cool to use a gravy for meats.

Per Cup: Calories: 112; Fat: 2g; Carbohydrates: 5g; Phosphorus: 139mg; Potassium: 50mg ; Sodium: 44mg; Protein: 9g

CHEESE SAUCE

SERVES 5 / PREP TIME: 5 MINUTES / COOK TIME: 20 MINUTES

Great with pastas, lasagna or over white fish.

1/4 CUP ALL PURPOSE WHITE FLOUR

4 OZ CREAM CHEESE

1/2 CUP BRIE

3/4 CUP 1% LOW-FAT MILK/RICE MILK
(UNENRICHED)

1 TBSP BUTTER

1/4 TSP WHITE PEPPER

1 TSP BLACK PEPPER

1. Heat saucepan on a medium heat.
2. Add the butter to the pan on the side nearest to the handle.
3. Tilt the pan towards you and allow butter to melt, whilst trying not to let it cover the rest of the pan.
4. Now add the flour to the opposite side of the pan and gradually mix the flour into the butter - continue to mix until smooth.
5. Add the milk and stir thoroughly for 10 minutes until lumps dissolve.
6. Add the cheese (optional) and stir for a further 5 minutes.
7. Turn off the heat and serve immediately.

Per serving: Calories: 156; Fat: 12g; Carbohydrates: 9g; Phosphorus: 80mg; Potassium: 49mg ; Sodium: 87mg; Protein: 4g

CRANBERRY SAUCE

SERVES 2 / PREP TIME: NA / COOK TIME: 30 MINUTES

Great as a dip, with curries or even as a salad topper.

---

2 CUPS CRANBERRIES

1 CUP WATER

1 TSP RED WINE VINEGAR

1/2 LIME, JUICED

---

1. Add the ingredients to a pot over a high heat and bring to the boil.
2. Turn down the heat and allow to simmer for 20-30 minutes or until fruits have softened.
3. Keep an eye on water levels to ensure fruit does not dry out and burn.
4. Once soft, allow to cool slightly and blend in a food processor until smooth.
5. Add a pinch of salt/pepper to balance out the sweetness of the cranberries.

Per serving: Calories: 51; Fat: 0g; Carbohydrates: 13g; Phosphorus: 20mg; Potassium: 90mg ; Sodium: 2mg; Protein: 9g

CAJUN BLEND

SERVES 2 / PREP TIME: 5 MINUTES / COOK TIME: NA

Great as a dip, with curries or even as a salad topper.

---

1 GARLIC CLOVE, MINCED

2 TSP BLACK PEPPER

2 TSP CAYENNE PEPPER

1 TSP CHILI POWDER

2 TSP DRIED THYME

2 TSP DRIED OREGANO

---

1. Mix all ingredients together and store in an airtight container in a dry place.
2. Use as a rub for meats and fishes before cooking.

Per serving: Calories: 25; Fat: 1g; Carbohydrates: 5g; Phosphorus: 20mg; Potassium: 159mg ; Sodium: 112mg; Protein: 1g

DRY HERB RUB

SERVES 2 / PREP TIME: 5 MINUTES / COOK TIME: NA

Add to meats, vegetables and fish before cooking or add to a little oil to use as a marinade.

1 TSP BLACK PEPPER	1 TSP DRIED BASIL
1 GARLIC CLOVE, MINCED	1 TSP DRIED THYME
1 CELERY STALK, MINCED	1 TSP DRIED OREGANO
2 TSP MUSTARD SEEDS, CRUSHED	

1. Combine all ingredients in a food processor until a fine powder is formed.
2. Store in an airtight container in a dry place.
3. When ready to use, mix with 1 tbsp olive oil and baste meats/fish/vegetables or alternatively use as a dry rub for broiling.

Per serving: Calories: 25; Fat: 0g; Carbohydrates: 1g; Phosphorus: 1mg; Potassium: 30mg ; Sodium: 4mg; Protein: 0g

SPINACH PESTO

SERVES 2 / PREP TIME: 5 MINUTES / COOK TIME: NA

Delicious kidney friendly pesto!

1/2 CUP FRESH BASIL

1/2 CUP FRESH SPINACH

1 TSP BLACK PEPPER

1/4 CUP EXTRA VIRGIN OLIVE OIL

1 GARLIC CLOVE, MINCED

1 LEMON, JUICED

---

1. Blend all ingredients in a food processor or a blender to reach required texture - chunky for a rustic feel or smooth as a dressing.
2. Store in an airtight container in the fridge for 3-4 days.
3. Serve over pasta, roasted vegetables, or as a dip for your favorite raw veg!

Per serving: Calories: 59; Fat: 0g; Carbohydrates: 0g; Phosphorus: 7mg; Potassium: 107mg ; Sodium: 56mg; Protein: 0g

DRINKS AND DESSERTS

BRILLIANT BERRY SMOOTHIE

SERVES 2 / PREP TIME: 5 MINUTES / COOK TIME: NA

Healthy strawberry milkshake that everyone can enjoy!

1/4 CUP STRAWBERRIES, SLICED

1/4 CUP BLUEBERRIES

1/4 CUP BLACKBERRIES

1 CUP RICE MILK, UNENRICHED

---

1. Blend in a food processor or smoothie maker and serve over ice if desired.
2. Enjoy!

Per serving: Calories: 90; Fat: 1g; Carbohydrates: 18g; Phosphorus: 82mg; Potassium: 70mg ; Sodium: 30mg; Protein: 1g

ANTIOXIDANT SMOOTHIES

SERVES 2 / PREP TIME: 5 MINUTES / COOK TIME: NA

This delectable smoothie is full of powerful antioxidants.

1/2 CUP RED OR WHITE GRAPES

1/2 CUP SLICED FROZEN OR FRESH PEACHES

1/2 CUP CHOPPED CABBAGE

1/4 CUP ICE CUBES

1/4 CUP WATER

1 SPRIG OF FRESH MINT

---

1. Toss all of the ingredients in a blender or juicer and blend until smooth.
2. Serve immediately in tall glasses.
3. Tear mint with fingers and serve with smoothies (optional).

Per serving: Calories: 48; Fat: 0g; Carbohydrates: 12g; Phosphorus: 17mg; Potassium: 203mg ; Sodium: 6mg; Protein: 1g

PANCAKES WITH PEACHES

SERVES 2 / PREP TIME: 5 MINUTES / COOK TIME: 10 MINUTES

Great for your sweet tooth!

---

2 FREE RANGE EGG WHITES

2 TBSP ALL PURPOSE WHITE FLOUR

3 TBSP COCONUT SHAVINGS

2 TBSP COCONUT MILK (OPTIONAL)

1 TBSP COCONUT OIL

1/2 CUP PEACHES, SLICED

---

1. Get a bowl and combine all the ingredients.
2. Mix well until you get a thick batter.
3. Heat a skillet on a medium heat and heat the coconut oil.
4. Pour half the mixture to the center of the pan, forming a pancake and cook through for 3-4 minutes on each side.
5. Serve with sliced peaches (you can warm these through in a skillet for 5 minutes if you wish).

Per serving: Calories: 425; Fat: 35g; Carbohydrates: 17g; Phosphorus: 85mg; Potassium: 150mg ; Sodium: 75mg; Protein: 10g

SPICED PEARS

SERVES 2 / PREP TIME: 5 MINUTES / COOK TIME: 10 MINUTES

A warming winter pudding.

---

1 CUP CANNED PEARS IN THEIR OWN JUICES

1/2 TSP CORNSTARCH

1 TSP GROUND CLOVES

1 TSP GROUND CINNAMON

1 TSP GROUND NUTMEG

ZEST OF 1/2 LEMON

1/2 CUP WATER

---

1. Drain pears.
2. Combine water cornstarch, , cinnamon, nutmeg, ground cloves and lemon zest in a pan on the stove.
3. Heat on a medium heat and add pears.
4. Bring to a boil, reduce the heat and simmer for 10 minutes.
5. Serve warm.

Per serving: Calories: 112; Fat: 0g; Carbohydrates: 25g; Phosphorus: 21mg; Potassium: 105mg ; Sodium: 7mg; Protein: 0g

MINI RASPBERRY MUFFINS

SERVES 2 / PREP TIME: 10 MINUTES / COOK TIME: 35 MINUTES

These are delicious served with extra fresh fruit or on their own.

---

1 1/2 EGG WHITES

1/8 CUP ALL PURPOSE WHITE FLOUR

1 TSP COCONUT FLOUR

1 TSP NUTMEG, GRATED

1 TSP VANILLA EXTRACT

1 TSP STEVIA

1/4 CUP FRESH RASPBERRIES

---

1. Pre-heat the oven to 325°F/170 °C/Gas Mark 3.
2. Mix all of the ingredients in a mixing bowl.
3. Divide the batter into 4 and spoon into a lightly oiled muffin tin.
4. Bake in the oven for 15-20 minutes or until cooked through.
5. Your knife should pull out clean from the middle of the muffin once done.
6. Allow to cool on a wired rack before serving.

Per serving: Calories: 97; Fat: 2g; Carbohydrates: 12g; Phosphorus: 72mg; Potassium: 65mg ; Sodium: 62mg; Protein: 4g

CONVERSION TABLES

Volume

Imperial	Metric
1 tbsp	15ml
2 fl oz	55 ml
3 fl oz	75 ml
5 fl oz (¼ pint)	150 ml
10 fl oz (½ pint)	275 ml
1 pint	570 ml
1 ¼ pints	725 ml
1 ¾ pints	1 litre
2 pints	1.2 litres
2½ pints	1.5 litres
4 pints	2.25 litres

Oven temperatures

Gas Mark	Fahrenheit	Celsius
1/4	225	110
1/2	250	130
1	275	140
2	300	150
3	325	170
4	350	180
5	375	190
6	400	200
7	425	220
8	450	230
9	475	240

Weight

Imperial	Metric
½ oz	10 g
¾ oz	20 g
1 oz	25 g
1½ oz	40 g
2 oz	50 g
2½ oz	60 g
3 oz	75 g
4 oz	110 g
4½ oz	125 g
5 oz	150 g
6 oz	175 g
7 oz	200 g
8 oz	225 g
9 oz	250 g
10 oz	275 g

BIBLIOGRAPHY

Garrick, R. (2008) 'Prevalence of chronic kidney disease in the United States', Yearbook of Medicine, 2008, pp. 215–217. doi: 10.1016/s0084-3873(08)79151-x.

Coresh, J., Astor, B.C., Greene, T., Eknoyan, G. and Levey, A.S. (2003) 'Prevalence of chronic kidney disease and decreased kidney function in the adult US population: Third national health and nutrition examination survey', American Journal of Kidney Diseases, 41(1), pp. 1–12. doi: 10.1053/ajkd.2003.50007.

Kopple, J.D. (2001) 'National kidney foundation K/DOQI clinical practice guidelines for nutrition in chronic renal failure', American Journal of Kidney Diseases, 37(1), pp. S66–S70. doi: 10.1053/ajkd.2001.20748.

Wilhelm-Leen, E.R., Hall, Y.N., Tamura, M.K. and Chertow, G.M. (2009) 'Frailty and chronic kidney disease: The Third national health and nutrition evaluation survey', The American Journal of Medicine, 122(7), pp. 664–671.e2. doi: 10.1016/j.amjmed.2009.01.026

Kidney Disease Outcomes Quality Initiative (K/DOQI) and the Dialysis Outcomes and Practice Patterns Study (DOPPS): Nutrition guidelines, indicators, and practices

Kalantar-Zadeh, K., Gutekunst, L., Mehrotra, R., Kovesdy, C.P., Bross, R., Shinaberger, C.S., Noori, N., Hirschberg, R., Benner, D., Nissenson, A.R. and Kopple, J.D. (2010) 'Understanding sources of dietary phosphorus in the treatment of patients with chronic kidney disease', Clinical Journal of the American Society of Nephrology, 5(3), pp. 519–530. doi: 10.2215/cjn.06080809.

Epstein, F.H., Brenner, B.M., Meyer, T.W. and Hostetter, T.H. (1982) 'Dietary protein intake and the progressive nature of kidney disease:', New England Journal of Medicine, 307(11), pp. 652–659. doi: 10.1056/nejm198209093071104.

Research, K. (2016) Kidney research UK - kidney research UK. Available at: https://www.kidneyresearchuk.org/health-information/chronic-kidney-disease (Accessed: 25 March 2016).

Foundation, N.K. (2014) Nutrition. Available at: https://www.kidney.org/nutrition (Accessed: 20 February2016).

nc, D.H.P. (2004) Top 15 healthy foods for people with kidney disease. Available at: https://www.davita.com/kidney-disease/diet-and-nutrition/lifestyle/top-15-healthy-foods-for-people-with-kidney-disease/e/5347 (Accessed: 25 July 2016).

INDEX

www.ingramcontent.com/pod-product-compliance
Lightning Source LLC
Chambersburg PA
CBHW051342200326

41521CB00015B/2586